The
Obesity
Myth

For my daughter, Leia

The
Obesity
Myth

Why America's Obsession with Weight
Is Hazardous to Your Health

PAUL CAMPOS

GOTHAM BOOKS
Published by Penguin Group (USA) Inc., 375 Hudson Street,
New York, New York 10014, U.S.A.
Penguin Books Ltd, Registered Offices: 80 Strand, London WC2R 0RL, England
Penguin Books Australia Ltd, 250 Camberwell Road, Camberwell, Victoria 3124, Australia
Penguin Books Canada Ltd, 10 Alcorn Avenue, Toronto, Ontario, Canada M4V 3B2
Penguin Books (NZ) cnr Airborne and Rosedale Roads,
Albany, Auckland 1310, New Zealand

Published by Gotham Books, a division of Penguin Group (USA) Inc.

First printing, May 2004
10   9   8   7   6   5   4   3   2   1

Excerpt from "Let Them Eat Fat: The Heavy Truths About American Obesity"
by Greg Critser, reprinted with permission from *Harper's* magazine.

LIBRARY OF CONGRESS CATALOGING-IN-PUBLICATION DATA
has been applied for.

ISBN: 1-592-40066-3

Printed in the United States of America
Set in Fairfield
Designed by Sabrina Bowers

Contents

Part III: Fat Politics

Foreword

THE WAVE OF HYSTERIA surrounding obesity can be traced back to many watershed events. In 1986, an NIH consensus panel on obesity ignored nearly all of the data presented to it and declared obesity a serious health threat. It did so despite presentations showing that people who gained weight as they aged reduced their risk of premature death, and that obesity was not related to hardening of the arteries. In the press conference afterward, the panel went much further and declared obesity to be a "a killer disease." This idea did not catch on at that time, even among anti-fat crusaders. In the early 1990s a more moderate and balanced view of obesity prevailed, illustrated by congressional hearings that found fault with the weight-loss industry and emphasized the mild nature of obesity-associated risks for all but the most extreme cases.

I recall vividly the day I realized that obesity science was out of control and out of touch with reality. It was at the 1996 FDA hearing on the approval of dexfenfluramine, the most damaging half of the wildly popular drug regimen known as fen-phen. The fen-phen craze was triggered by publication of a single small trial of the drug combination in 1992, conducted by John Weintraub. Few people knew it then, but the publication costs were paid by the drug's manufacturers. Weintraub was hired by the FDA, and continued to promote the drug combination while he was an FDA employee. Clinics devoted to writing prescriptions for fen-phen, and collecting fat fees from them, were springing up all over the country. The major diet clinic chains like Nutri-System were offering fen-phen prescriptions in their store-fronts. A big obstacle to promotion of these diet pills, however, was that their use was strictly limited to twelve weeks. Use beyond this time was thought to be too dangerous because of side effects and the potential for addiction. So the drug's manufacturer sought approval for a reformulation of fenfluramine—known as dexfenfluramine or Redux—intended for lifelong use. Editorials by obesity experts duly appeared, calling for lifelong use of diet pills, and comparing obesity to chronic conditions, such as high blood pressure, that need daily treat-ment for life. George Bray, a leading expert, famously quipped, "Drugs don't work when not taken," implying that one needed to take diet pills permanently to achieve permanent weight loss.

When I arrived to testify at the FDA hearing that would decide dexfenfluramine's fate, I was struck by the impressive array of obesity experts in attendance. Everyone who was anyone seemed to be there. I was there, in part, because experiments with laboratory animals con-ducted by my colleagues and me at Case Western Reserve University indicated that regaining lost weight undoes all of the apparent benefits of weight loss, and also creates new problems, such as high blood pres-sure, enlargement of the heart, and even kidney damage. Indeed, long-term human studies show that almost all of the excess risk associated with obesity can be accounted for by the higher incidence of weight cycling in obese people, and that obese people with stable weights have very little excess risk.

George Bray came over and greeted me, and I expressed my awe at the assemblage of experts. "This is an important day for the obesity field," he said loftily. "We are all united in our support for this drug ap-proval," he said a bit pointedly, knowing that I was about to testify against approval. I wasn't the least bit shaken. I was well aware that in the past the obesity field had been just as impressively united be-hind many failed treatments, including intestinal bypass surgery, zero-calorie diets, liquid-protein diets, jaw wiring, thyroid pills, injections of horse urine extract, and amphetamines. As a scientific (as opposed to an economic) matter, obesity research did not have an impressive record of success—and it was about to get worse. A simple computer search using the words "fenfluramine" and "adverse effect" turned up hundreds of reports. The drug was already linked to a fatal lung condition in people, and to brain damage in animals. Rarely, if ever, had a drug with such a long history of dangerous side effects been up for government approval. And for what benefit? The clinical data indicated that dieters taking fenfluramine lost only seven pounds more than dieters taking a placebo. As I testified to the FDA committee, this was not a favorable ratio of risk to benefit. There is a gradual fall of life expectancy associated with extremes of weight, resulting ultimately in a loss of six to eight years of life expectancy for "morbidly obese" women. In other words, being 150 pounds "overweight" has a risk association similar to that seen with light cigarette smoking. But a loss of seven pounds would not move anyone perceptibly down this risk gradient. More important, dexfenfluramine had not been shown to produce any improvement whatsoever in the major risk factors associated with high weight, such as blood pressure and cholesterol. It is these risk factors that form the rationale for treating obesity in the first place, so why approve a drug that had no proven health benefit other than producing a tiny amount of weight loss?

My testimony was followed by that of Judith Stern, professor of nutrition at the University of California–Davis. She testified that she was speaking not as an expert but rather simply "as an obese woman" who wanted to see a "valuable" treatment made available. She spoke on behalf of the American Obesity Association, a powerful DC lobbying group, funded by drug companies and the diet industry, that claims to represent the interests of 160 million "overweight" Americans. After the hearing, she told the Associated Press that any expert who opposed approval of Redux "should be shot." Clearly, emotions were running high among obesity experts, many of whom were eager to keep their pill-dispensing clinics open and filled with patients desperate to lose weight.

Further key testimony came from Jo Ann Manson of the Harvard Medical School. She did not dispute the fact that the drug had fatal side effects and produced an average weight loss of only seven pounds. But she argued that extra weight was so deadly that a seven-pound weight loss would save slightly more lives than would be lost from the fatal lung disease caused by the drug. She assumed a great many things in making this argument, some of which seem especially absurd in retrospect. For example, she assumed that 100% of the side effects

of the drug had been noted by physicians, that 100% of these side effects had been reported to the drug company, and that 100% of these
reports had been passed along immediately to the FDA. Note that in
the case of the fatal lung disease (primary pulmonary hypertension),
the only symptom may be shortness of breath. How many obese people are short of breath? Typically, patients can go years with these
symptoms before a diagnosis is made, if indeed it is ever made. And, if
the patient dies, it is all too common for obesity to be blamed, rather
than the diet pills the patient was taking. Busy physicians report only
a fraction of adverse drug reactions to the manufacturer, and usually
only in those cases where the adverse reactions can't be blamed on
another cause, such as obesity. Nevertheless Manson's fanciful interpretation of the data, which attributed life-saving benefits to an average weight loss of seven pounds, appeared to be highly convincing to
the FDA panel, as revealed by the discussions preceding the vote for
approval.

I had pictured an FDA hearing as a sort of trial, with the drug company as the defense attorney, the FDA taking the role of prosecutor,
and the expert medical panel playing the part of the jury. Instead, the
FDA and Wyeth (the drug's manufacturer) formed a team that tried to
persuade the panel to approve the drug. It fell to a panel of academic
physicians, none of them specially trained in pharmacology, to try to
find the weaknesses in the FDA's and Wyeth's joint advocacy, and
to ask the right questions about the risks of serious and/or fatal side
effects.

We all know the aftermath. Even though fenfluramine and dexfenfluramine were taken off the market in 1997, millions of patients have
heart damage as a consequence of taking these pills, and continue to
be monitored by cardiologists. Billions of dollars have been paid out by
the manufacturers in wrongful death and injury lawsuits. Were the
obesity experts chastened by these events? Did they adopt a more cau-
tious approach toward promoting obesity treatments? The opposite
seems to have happened. Despite the absence of any safe and effective treatment for obesity, ineffective and dangerous treatments continue to be promoted relentlessly. Another diet pill with potentially
dangerous side effects, sibutramine (Meridia), was approved by the
same FDA panel despite evidence that it raises blood pressure and

that it may be linked to strokes. The Center for Science in the Public Interest has petitioned the FDA to withdraw its approval, and sales were temporarily suspended in Europe after a series of deaths in young women taking the drug. And so it goes.

The fen-phen scandal did chasten the major medical journals. Jo Ann Manson published her FDA testimony as an editorial in the *New England Journal of Medicine*, which argued again that even though dexfenfluramine had fatal side effects, seven pounds of weight loss justified the risk and expense of taking the drug. The editorial was a rebuttal to an epidemiological study showing that dexfenfluramine increased the risk of fatal lung disease by 2,300%. There was no indication that Manson and her co-author had financial links to the drug maker—a circumstance that played a part in the subsequent tightening of conflict-of-interest rules for many medical journals.

Although it might seem obvious, it needs to be said that drugs and other treatments should only be used when they have clear benefits to health, not simply because they produce weight loss—and that furthermore, those benefits must exceed the accompanying risks. After all, smoking crack cocaine is an effective way to reduce body weight, but I doubt most obesity experts would recommend employing it as a weight-loss treatment. Yet in the current climate of hysteria over obesity, both our public health establishment and the public it counsels seem increasingly willing to accept grave risks and steep costs in exchange for small and usually temporary losses of body mass. Where will it end?

In this book, Paul Campos examines the current media frenzy surrounding weight and weight-loss issues. He delves into the realm of statistics and epidemiology to explore the foundations for this rising tide of fear and loathing surrounding body fat, and finds little or no scientific basis for that fear, except in regard to the small minority of people who are at the extremes of body weight: the very thin and the very fat. He explores the cultural sources of our current panic over weight, and discovers the fingerprints of a multibillion-dollar weight loss industry at every turn. But rather than pointing to medical-industrial conspiracies, he identifies long-standing cultural and social trends as the underlying forces that fuel the obesity myth. In lively yet erudite prose, Campos treats the obesity debate as a trial, where fat is the defendant, the obesity industry is the prosecutor, and we are the jury. In doing so, he provides us with an entertaining and enlightening treatment of a topic that for too long has been the subject of fear-driven hysteria, rather than rational debate.

—Paul Ernsberger, Ph.D.

Introduction

IS YOUR WEIGHT hazardous to your health? According to America's public health authorities, there's an 80% chance that it is. From the Surgeon General's office, the Centers for Disease Control, the National Institutes of Health, and our leading medical schools, America's anti-fat warriors are bombarding us with dire warnings: According to such sources, no less than four of every five Americans maintain a medically dangerous body mass (nearly two-thirds of us are said to be overweight, while almost half of the rest of the nation is categorized as too thin).

If these claims sound implausible, there's a very good reason why: because they're false. Indeed, given that Americans are enjoying longer lives and better health than ever before, the claim that four out of five of us are running serious health risks because of our weight sounds exactly like the sort of exaggeration that can produce a cultural epidemic of fear, bearing no relation to any rational assessment of risk.

On the other hand, given the pervasiveness of America's fear of fat, it's only natural that many readers will react skeptically to a claim that this fear has no real medical or scientific justification. For one thing, it is always disturbing to acknowledge that authoritative social institutions can and sometimes do seriously mislead the public: At some level everyone would like to be able to trust our culture's experts and authority figures when they claim to know what's best for us. Indeed, when I began researching this topic five years ago, I assumed the fact that being "overweight" was a serious health risk was so well established that this aspect of the subject was hardly worth discussing. Yet in the course of plowing through dozens of books, hundreds of articles in medical journals, and countless interviews with medical and scientific experts, I discovered that almost everything the government and the media were saying about weight and weight control was either grossly distorted or flatly untrue.

What I discovered was that a host of eminent doctors, scientists, eating disorder specialists, psychologists, sociologists, and other critics of America's obsession with weight and weight loss have concluded that "overweight" and "obesity" are not primarily medical issues at all. In the wake of a century's worth of unsuccessful attempts to find a cure for the "disease" of a higher-than-average weight, a diverse and distinguished group of critics has come to see weight in America as primarily a cultural and political issue. Indeed these opponents of the war on fat have subjected the supposed medical justifications for that war to devastating criticisms. Such critics point out that there is nothing new about either America's "obesity epidemic," or the public health warnings it inspires. For more than fifty years now, government officials have been making the same dire predictions concerning the public health calamity that is about to befall us as a consequence of the nation's expanding waistline (as long ago as the 1950s, nearly half of America's adult population was supposedly overweight).

One goal of this book is to make it clear that several decades' worth of grim prophecies regarding the devastating health consequences of higher-than-average weight have turned out to be spectacularly inaccurate. Another is to explicitly politicize what in fact is a political issue, by expanding America's public debate about weight and weight control to include the opinions of people who do not run weight loss clinics. This isn't a rhetorical exaggeration: It has become routine for government panels charged with the task of making public health recommendations regarding weight to consist exclusively of people who run weight loss clinics.

As a lawyer I thought I had become accustomed to the extent to which people are willing to bend, spindle, and mutilate the truth in the pursuit of their own interests. But nothing could have prepared me for the sheer extent of the distortions that feed America's rapidly intensifying weight hysteria. (Consider that a search of the major media for stories regarding the "obesity epidemic" reveals a twentyfold increase in such stories over the course of the last five years.) This book documents how the current barrage of claims about the supposedly devastating medical and economic consequences of "excess" weight is a product of greed, junk science, and outright bigotry. It blows the whistle on a witch-hunt masquerading as a public health initiative, by exposing the invidious cultural forces that encourage us to hate our bodies if they fail to conform to an arbitrary and absurdly restrictive ideal. And it outlines how we can begin to embrace a saner definition of what constitutes a healthy lifestyle and a desirable body.

I began working on this project, in part, because I suspected a well-known critic of the war on fat (Richard Klein) was on to something when he pointed to "a growing awareness that the whole culture of dieting and rigid exercise is the root cause of the fat explosion." I have since discovered that, as disturbingly accurate as that insight into the perverse paradox at the heart of the war on fat was, the damage wrought by this war goes far beyond its tendency to expand our waistlines. Historically most attempts to marginalize and shame some disfavored class of people have focused on minority groups of one sort or another. The war on fat is unique in American history in that it represents the first concerted attempt to transform the vast majority of the nation's citizens into social pariahs, to be pitied and scorned until weapons of mass destruction can be found that will rid them of their shameful condition. As we shall see, this is a phony war, fought against an enemy that cannot be defeated, because he does not exist.

The rejection of the war on fat is based on a simple principle: that tolerance toward an almost wholly benign form of human diversity is the least we should expect of ourselves, if we wish to lay claim to living in a civilized culture. The war on fat is an outrage to values—of equality, of tolerance, of fairness, and indeed of fundamental decency toward those who are different—that American culture celebrates (often with good reason) as essential features of our nation's character. And in the end nothing could be easier than to win this war: All we need to do is stop fighting it.

The war on fat has especially devastating consequences for women. Indeed, I'm not sure I've ever met an American woman who genuinely likes her body. I don't doubt there are such women in contemporary

xviii   INTRODUCTION

America (especially among ethnic minority groups). Still, after having interviewed hundreds of women regarding their feelings about food, fat, body image, and what it's like to deal with these issues in America today, I can't say I'm confident I've actually encountered such a person.

The stories these women would tell were always sad, sometimes harrowing, and often appalling. Some of them have been included in this book. I wish I could have included many more: Recently, a young woman from what is considered a privileged background recounted to me, in the course of describing the weight hysteria that dominated the milieu in which she was raised, how a girl she grew up with was never permitted to go on a date without first being weighed by her father. If the number on the scale was too high, she was forced to go jogging before her date arrived.

We live in a culture that tells the average American woman, dozens of times per day, that the shape of her body is the most important thing about her, and that she should be disgusted by it. How can one begin to calculate the full emotional, financial, and physiological toll exacted by such messages? And although women pay the highest price for our national obsession with weight, the cultural hysteria regarding this subject is becoming so intense that, increasingly, men are beginning to show signs of the damage that is done to people when they are told constantly that there is something fundamentally wrong with them.

Whether we are supposedly too fat, or too thin, or too sedentary, or too prone to eat unhealthy food, our medical and governmental authorities never tire of hectoring Americans about our imperfections. Between, on the one hand, our punitive public health nannies, and, on the other, the entrepreneurs who hawk health club memberships, workout equipment, Botox, Viagra, and dozens of similar drugs, as well as thousands of varieties of cosmetics, various sorts of plastic surgery, and most of all a seemingly unlimited parade of diets, each of which promises us the illusion of perpetual youth in the guise of slenderness, we have constructed a culture that ensures that relatively few people will ever be at peace with their bodies.

In America today the medical and public health establishment has managed to transform what has traditionally been considered a vice—physical vanity—into that most sacred of secular virtues: the pursuit of "health." In the context of the war on fat it has done so by systematically distorting the available evidence regarding the relationship between weight and health, by severely exaggerating the risks associated with that evidence, and by pretending that an extremely complex subject is actually quite simple.

These are harsh charges, but if anything, they understate the scandal that is the war on fat. Never before in American history has so much junk science been exploited to whip up hysteria about a supposed public health "epidemic." The health establishment's constant barrage of scientifically baseless propaganda regarding the relationship between weight and health constitutes nothing less than egregious abuse of the public trust. This propaganda has played a key role in creating a culture that makes tens of millions of people miserable about their bodies. Worse yet, it has done so for crass economic motives. The war on fat, which is supposedly about making all of us healthy, is really about making some of us rich.

Yet, as we shall see, the sources of America's weight loss mania go well beyond the fact that the dietary-pharmaceutical complex finds it profitable to nurture and exploit our national obsession with thinness. It is no exaggeration to say that in many respects contemporary America is a fundamentally eating-disordered culture. A much-noted sign of this can be seen in the binge-sized portions that are now standard fare in our restaurants and fast-food emporia. A less-noted piece of evidence is provided by the almost overtly anorexic quality of much of the current hysteria about fat. One explanation for the remarkable distortions of the medical evidence in which those who prosecute the case against fat indulge is that many of these people see that evidence through anorexic eyes. Let me be clear: I am not claiming that all such persons are technically anorexic (although some undoubtedly are). What I am saying is that the anorexic mindset is far more common than our narrow definition of what constitutes instances of the syndrome itself, and that this mindset has played an important part in producing America's growing intolerance of even the mildest forms of body diversity.

Consider that anyone who attends a conference on the "obesity epidemic" in America today is likely to find that a good number of the participants are extremely thin, high-achieving, upper-class white women, many of whom appear to have both strong perfectionist tendencies and a pathological fear and loathing of fat. Any accurate account of the war on fat must grapple with the fact that many obesity researchers, eating disorder specialists, nutritionists, etc., belong to the precise social groups that are at the highest risk for anorexia nervosa—and that indeed a significant number of these individuals display at least some of the classic symptoms of the syndrome. For example, by some estimates, an actual majority of dietitians either have or have had eating disorders. It is true that, to the extent such persons have both recovered from and come to terms with their eating disorders, their backgrounds can improve the quality of their work. But it is also clear that large numbers of people who make it their professional business to counsel Americans about weight and health remain either actively eating disordered, or prone to the same patterns of thinking that fuel such behaviors. In short, much of the advice Americans get about weight can be compared to getting advice about drinking from people who are alcoholics and don't know it.

What, after all, leads medical authorities to conclude that a 146-pound woman of average height is "overweight"? Beyond the fact that it's economically profitable to classify her as fat, we should remember that, for those in the grip of what the eating disorders literature calls "anorexic ideation" (i.e., the tendency to interpret the world through an anorexic lens), a 146-pound woman *is* fat. Indeed, some obesity researchers are now recommending that the body "ideal" should be redefined to exclude anyone with a body mass index above 21.9—a definition that would make a 128-pound woman of average height "fat."

Such recommendations, I would suggest, are the natural consequences of allowing persons who see the world through anorexic eyes to define what "normal" means. On one level, this claim shouldn't even be controversial: After all, it's now routine to acknowledge that the stick-thin models and movie stars who are held up for emulation to America and the world are quite literally images of an anorexic ideal.

Why is there so little outrage over this? Anorexia nervosa has by far the highest fatality rate of any mental illness; eight million Americans are estimated to be suffering from eating disorders; tens of millions of others regularly engage in disordered eating of some sort; and yet somehow, the fact that much of American culture—from the sound stages of Hollywood to the office of the Surgeon General—is in the grip of an anorexic worldview is something that is more or less taken for granted.

For too long, too few people have been willing to condemn that view for being the destructive distortion of reality that it is. This book is for everyone who lives with the daily consequences of the lies that an eating-disordered culture tells them about their bodies. It is for everyone who has been told they are too fat—or too thin. It's for everyone who has been encouraged to believe the propaganda of our public health authorities, instead of listening to the truth being told to them by their own bodies: that living a joyful, active life—one that includes the calm enjoyment of the many pleasures afforded by food—promotes health and longevity, while trying to conform to some arbitrary body "ideal" does damage to both.

To the tens of millions of Americans who are being made miserable by the lies of the weight loss industry, and its mouthpieces in the medical and public health establishments, I would say this: Rejecting those lies requires nothing less than an act of personal and social revolt. And nothing less than a revolution is needed to overthrow America's eating-disordered culture, with its loathing of the most minimal body diversity, its neurotic oscillation between guilt-ridden bingeing and anorexic self-starvation, and its pathological fear of food, pleasure, and life itself.

Indeed, our whole diet culture is ultimately all about fear, and self-loathing, and endless dissatisfaction. That is the culture we live in. That is the culture we must change. If you have spent much of your life hating your body, because you have been told over and over again that there is something wrong with it, this book will explain just how false that message is. And it will explain exactly what has gone wrong with a culture that demands you hate the body you were born with.

This book has three parts. Part I, "Fat Science," provides a concise overview of the current medical literature on the relationship between weight and health. Many of the facts in this section are likely to astonish anyone who has relied on the mass media for information on this topic (they certainly astonished me). Contrary to almost everything you have heard, weight is not a good predictor of health. In fact a moderately active larger person is likely to be far healthier than someone who is svelte but sedentary. Moreover, the efforts of Americans to make themselves thin through dieting and drugs are a major cause of both "overweight" and the ill health that is wrongly ascribed to it. In other words, America's war on fat is actually helping cause the very disease it is supposed to cure. In the chapters that follow, we will see that:

> ➤ The health risks associated with increasing weight are gener-
> ally small, in comparison to those associated with, for example,
> being a man, or poor, or African American.

> ➤ These risks tend to disappear altogether when factors other
> than weight are taken into account. For instance, fat active
> people have half the mortality rate of thin sedentary people,
> and the same mortality rate as thin active people.

> ➤ There is no good evidence that significant long-term weight
> loss is beneficial to health, and a great deal of evidence that
> short-term weight loss followed by weight regain (the pattern
> followed by almost all dieters) is medically harmful. Indeed,
> frequent dieting is perhaps the single best predictor of future
> weight gain.

> ➤ Despite a century-long search for a "cure" for "overweight," we
> still have no idea how to make fat people thin.

As this part of the book will make clear, the war on fat has reached
the point where systematic distortion of the evidence has become the
norm, rather than the exception. The basic strategies employed by
those who profit from this war are to treat the most extreme cases as
typical, to ignore all contrary data, and to recommend "solutions" that
actually cause the problems they supposedly address. And, as in all
wars, truth ends up being the first casualty.

To a shocking extent, much of the highest profile obesity research
being done in America today turns out to be little more than propaganda masquerading as the results of disinterested scientific investigation: propaganda that has been bought and paid for by our nation's
$50 billion per year weight loss industry. The book's first section illus-
trates the extent to which Americans have become as addicted to junk
science as we are to junk food—and it lays the groundwork for exploring that addiction's profound cultural and political consequences.

As we will see in Part II, "Fat Culture," the war on fat ultimately
has very little to do with science. The doctors and public health officials prosecuting that war would have us believe that who is or isn't fat
is a scientific question that can be answered by consulting something
as crude as a body mass index chart (the BMI is a simple mathematical formula that puts people of different heights and weights on a sin-

gle integrated scale). This, like so many other claims at the heart of the case against fat, is false. "Fat"—or as our anti-fat warriors prefer to put it, "overweight"—is a cultural construct, not a scientific fact. For instance, according to the public health establishment's current BMI definitions, Brad Pitt, Michael Jordan, and Mel Gibson are all "overweight," while Russell Crowe, George Clooney, and baseball star Sammy Sosa are all "obese." (A common reaction to such absurdities is to object that the BMI definitions aren't meant to apply to people in "good shape." In fact, those who make claims about the supposed link between increasing body mass and ill health do not make exceptions for movie stars, athletes, or anyone else. According to America's fat police, if your BMI is over 25 then you are "overweight," period. Note also the radical difference between how our culture defines "fashionable" thinness for men and women. If Jennifer Aniston had the same BMI as her husband Brad Pitt, she would weigh approximately 55 pounds more than she does.)

The truth is that to be fat in America today means to weigh more than whatever a person's particular social milieu considers appropriate. As we shall see, this means it is perfectly possible—and in a certain twisted sense even "reasonable"—for a 130-pound white college student of average height to consider herself "fat," while a working-class African American woman who weighs 50 pounds more is not likely to think of herself as "overweight" (and she, too, will be correct in her self-assessment). In other words, fat in America is a state of mind, rather than some objective fact about our bodies.

Although race and class are topics that make most Americans nearly as uncomfortable as fat itself, any extensive discussion of weight-related issues must explore the many connections between these three subjects. "Fat Culture" outlines how such disparate topics as Gwyneth Paltrow's fat suit, Michael Jackson's attempts to become white, Elvis Presley's expanding waistline, the "food porn" of high-end restaurant menu prose, and the kidnapping of a three-year-old girl by the state of New Mexico because she was "too fat" are all fundamentally interconnected.

Americans love to moralize about fat because, among other reasons, fat has become a convenient stand-in for various characteristics that have been traditionally associated with the pariahs of the moment. "Fat Culture" explores how and why Americans who would never dream of consciously allowing themselves to be disgusted by someone's skin color, or religion, or social class, often feel no compunction about expressing the disgust elicited in them by the sight of people who weigh anything from a lot to a little more than our current absurdly restrictive cultural ideal.

Such reactions are ultimately political in the broadest sense; and Part III, "Fat Politics," traces the political consequences of an ideology that equates thinness with virtue and fat with vice. Indeed this ideology drives both the science and culture of our national obsession with weight and weight control. This part of the book describes how that obsession came to play a key role in the impeachment of the president of the United States; and it explores the powerful political meanings and messages that Americans have come to ascribe to the shape of peoples' bodies. The argument in these chapters suggests that, for upper-class Americans in particular, obsessing about weight can become a way of dealing with (or rather not dealing with) far more significant issues involving consumption and overconsumption.

In American culture, the urge to moralize and medicalize as many aspects of personal behavior as possible runs deep. Today epidemiological regression analyses have largely taken the place of the sorts of exhortations once represented by Jonathan Edwards' eighteenth-century sermon "Sinners in the Hands of an Angry God." Nevertheless, as Part III will make clear, the motivating impulses behind such apparently dissimilar texts turn out to have a number of things in common. At bottom, the obesity myth is both a cause and a consequence of what sociologists call a "moral panic." It is a particularly tenacious example of the same sort of impulse that fueled hysteria about demon rum, reefer madness, communists in the State Department, witches in Salem, and many other instances of our eternally recurring search for scapegoats, who can be blamed for the decadent state of American culture in general, and of the younger generation in particular.

Our anti-fat warriors are right about one thing: How we approach issues of weight, weight control, and body image tells us a great deal about what kind of people we really are. Much like their Calvinist spiritual ancestors, those who prosecute the war on fat treat the most extreme forms of intolerance as the surest signs of virtue. And, as we shall see, in their unwillingness to brook dissent, their eagerness to sniff out heresy, and their ultimately tragic devotion to a task that can neither be completed nor abandoned, those who have transformed the Protestant work ethic into the American diet ethic are worthy heirs to a tradition of life-warping fanaticism.

Anyone who writes a book challenging the conventional wisdom on a controversial topic knows in advance that his arguments will be misunderstood, caricatured, and generally distorted by those who have the most to lose from the possibility that the challenge might be effective. Although it is futile to attempt to avoid that fate by anticipating it, it still might be useful to state a few points as clearly as possible from the outset, for the benefit of skeptical readers willing to consider the merits of this particular challenge.

The obesity myth is based on three claims: that "excess" weight causes illness and early death; that losing weight improves health and extends life; and that we know how to make fat people thin. It is true that these claims are not completely false. After all, as every good propagandist knows, a social myth is much more effective when it is based on a grain of truth.

This book does not argue that there is no relationship between weight and health. It argues, rather, that the health risks associated with higher-than-average weight have been greatly exaggerated, while all sorts of related but far graver risks have been ignored. In particular, this book emphasizes that poverty, poor nutrition, and a culture that makes it easy for Americans to be sedentary are important public health issues in America today. We should be encouraging Americans to be physically active, to eat well, and to provide reasonable access to medical care for those among us who lack it. What we should not be doing is telling Americans that they will improve their health by trying to lose weight. As we shall see, there is very little evidence that attempts to achieve weight loss will improve the health of most people who undertake them, and a great deal of evidence that such attempts do more harm than good.

Nevertheless, it's important to be realistic about the actual motivations that lead people to try to lose weight. This book acknowledges that, given the enormous premium our culture places on thinness, Americans have all sorts of reasons for wanting to lose weight that have nothing to do with health. But it also points out that treating cosmetic weight loss as if it were a medical and moral issue tends to make people both considerably fatter and a good deal unhappier than they would otherwise be.

Finally, it would be unfair to the reader not to reveal from the beginning that this book has an autobiographical dimension of a rather ironic sort. I lost a great deal of weight while working on this book, thereby transforming myself, in the course of undertaking a comprehensive critique of America's obsession with weight loss, from an "obese" forty-year-old man into someone who currently maintains what our public health establishment mischaracterizes as an "ideal" weight. I will explore the significance of this peculiar fact in the book's final chapter. For now I merely note that, given the dismal history of diets in America, it would only be fitting if the first really effective diet book consisted of a wholesale denunciation of the very idea of diet books. Indeed in the course of this project I discovered that there were distinct advantages to being a fat person hiding inside a thin body. Who, after all, can describe a prison more accurately than one of its inmates?

The
Obesity
Myth

PART I

FAT SCIENCE

Career science depends as much on career maneuvering, posturing, and politics as it does on research and the pursuit of the truth . . . The hardest thing I learned was that modern science does not welcome a truly new idea. And it makes mistakes even at the "self-evident" level of logic and math.

—BART KOSKO, *Fuzzy Logic*

I

Fat on Trial

IN THE WINTER OF 2003, as America prepared to go to war with Iraq, U.S. Surgeon General Richard Carmona warned the nation that it faced a far more dangerous threat than Saddam Hussein's weapons of mass destruction. Rather than focusing on the danger posed by nuclear, biological, and chemical weapons, Carmona told his audience, "Let's look at a threat that is very real, and already here: obesity." Carmona went on to recall a recent news conference at which reporters wanted to question him about national preparedness for dealing with terrorist attacks. "One of the reporters asked me, 'What is the most pressing issue in health facing the United States today?' " Carmona said. "She thought I was going to say weapons of mass destruction. But I said obesity. She was stunned. I mean, she couldn't say a word for thirty seconds because she didn't expect to hear 'obesity.' "

The reporter shouldn't have been surprised. Carmona is merely the latest in a series of Surgeon Generals who have treated America's expanding waistline as the nation's leading public health problem. From C. Everett Koop, who claimed that fat was killing one thousand Americans per day, to David Satcher—whose 2001 *Call to Action to Prevent and Decrease Overweight and Obesity* recommended that the government take immediate action to help "overweight" Americans lose weight—to Carmona himself—who believes that nearly two-thirds of us are too fat—America's leading public health spokesmen have been warning us for years that the nation faces a health crisis of cata-strophic proportions. In doing so, they have merely reflected the lan-guage of much of the medical establishment, which for many decades has treated "overweight" and "obesity" as major health risks. Medical researchers have gone so far as to recommend that high-fat and high-sugar foods be taxed to discourage people from eating them; and now, taking their cue from such warnings, enterprising lawyers are filing class-action suits against the fast-food industry, as in the wake of the tobacco litigation they seek other deep-pocket defendants on which to deploy their skills.

In America today fat is on trial. The case against fat is repeated al-most daily in the national media, in the form of stories that report the supposedly devastating effects of being "overweight," and which as-sure us that, if present trends go unchecked, everyone in America will be fat within another generation or so. If such a thing should come to pass, all of us, one supposes, will be eligible to become plaintiffs in the landmark class-action suit, *America v. Itself*, which will attempt to place the blame for this calamity on the appropriate villains.

What follows is an analysis of the evidence in the case against fat. The medical and public health establishment is telling the American people a seemingly straightforward story about the health risks of above-average weight, that comforts us because of the simplicity of its mes-sage (if you want to be healthy, stay or get thin). But the conventional wisdom regarding the relationship between weight and health distorts a far more complicated tale.

A question that might naturally arise in the minds of readers is: Why should a lawyer and law professor be arguing about this issue, rather than the doctors, nutritionists, and other scientists who make it their professional business to study these matters? One answer is that such people *have* been arguing about this issue for many decades now. Indeed, for much of the past century medical professionals have been disagreeing in the sharpest possible terms about whether the conven-tional wisdom regarding the relationship between weight and health is correct. Some of the most distinguished scholars in the field of obesity research argue not merely that the conventional wisdom is flawed: Rather, in their view, the case against fat is almost the precise opposite of the truth. Yet the broader public only rarely gets a glimpse of this ongoing debate. Fat is on trial, but until now the defense has been mostly absent from the court of public opinion. The reasons for that absence are themselves among the most interesting features of America's war on fat, and they too will be explored in this book.

But first things first: As the government continues to prosecute the case against fat, its indictment has gone, in the eyes of the public, largely unanswered. In these circumstances a lawyer is called for precisely because, in the court of public opinion (in sharp contrast to the arcane world of medical journals and professional conferences), the case has been so one-sided. Does this mean I am taking part in this controversy as an advocate for certain individuals or interest groups? No: I am an advocate for truth, and its indispensable partner, honesty—both of whom, as we shall see, have too often been barred from appearing in this particular trial.

The Case Against Fat

The simple story the medical and public health establishment tells the American public about the relationship between weight and health has three parts. The first and most basic part of the story could be labeled "Fat Kills." At bottom, the case against fat rests on the claim that the thinner you are, the longer you will live. The second part of the story is a narrative explaining why being thin is better for your health. We might call this narrative "Why Fat Is Deadly." The final part of the story tells Americans what to do with the information given them in parts one and two. It can be called "Get Thin." In what follows, I will describe the case against fat in the terms used by those who are most committed to the story outlined above. Then I will cross-examine that case in light of the actual evidence, to see how well it holds together when one does not simply assume that anything public health officials and medical authorities tell us must be true.

Fat Kills

For nearly a century now, the average American has been told that, if he or she wants to live longer, he or she should try to be thinner. Beginning with the Metropolitan Life Insurance tables devised in the 1940s, Americans have been assured that there is overwhelming statistical evidence for the proposition that people who are thinner than

average live longer than those who are not. Today the MetLife tables
have been largely superceded by the body mass index (BMI)—a simple mathematical formula that puts people of different heights and
weights on a single numerical scale (see the appendix for a BMI
chart). According to the latest BMI figures, 64.5% of American adults
are either "overweight" (meaning they have a BMI of between 25 and
29.9) or "obese" (defined as a BMI of 30 or higher). These definitions
are based on what Walter Willett and Meir Stampfer of the Harvard
School of Public Health call "a strong international consensus among
scientists that overweight (BMI over 25) and obesity are major contributors to morbidity and mortality." This belief in turn is based on
various epidemiological studies that demonstrate a correlation between
increasing body mass and premature death. As June Stevens, the author of one such study put it, "It's the very lean weight that is associated with the best survival rate."

Other studies have found an association between even mild amounts
of "overweight" and a significantly increased risk of premature death.
For example, a highly publicized study published in the *New England
Journal of Medicine* in 1995 found that women of average height who
were as little as 12 pounds overweight had a 60 percent increased risk
of mortality. A 1999 study published in the *Journal of the American Medical Association* estimated that overweight and obesity lead to
around three hundred thousand premature deaths per year in America
alone. The message the authors of such studies intend to convey is
clear: Excess weight will cost a large majority of today's Americans
years of life. The proportion of the population that maintains a dangerously high weight continues to climb: Obesity in America has increased by more than 50% over the course of the last decade alone. If
the authors of these studies are correct, America is facing a health crisis that, in the words of one anti-fat warrior, will make AIDS look "like
a bad case of the flu."

Why Fat Is Deadly

The National Institutes of Health (NIH) warn that being overweight
or obese "puts you at risk for developing many diseases, especially
heart disease, stroke, diabetes, and cancer." According to Yale Medical

School professor Kelly Brownell and Harvard Medical School professor David Ludwig, such risks make obesity an "epidemic [that] threatens the foundations of our society . . . To avert an impending calamity, public health must take precedence over private profit, action must replace apathy, and passiveness must give way to the protection of our children." Ludwig's colleague Walter Willett adds that "a wealth of literature" documents "powerful relationships between being overweight and the risks of coronary heart disease, diabetes, hypertension [and] various cancers." The Centers for Disease Control warn that overweight and obesity put persons at increased risk for congestive heart failure, coronary heart disease, diabetes, high blood pressure, obstructive sleep apnea and other respiratory problems, and some cancers.

The case against fat thus seems clear: Having a BMI of 25 (this is a weight of 146 pounds for a woman of average height, and 178 pounds for a man of average height) or higher has been proven by medical science to cause a myriad of deadly conditions. The question then becomes, what can we do about this epidemic that is dooming the more than 135 million adult Americans who are currently overweight to lives that, as a consequence of their excess weight, are likely to be marred by debilitating illness and early death?

Get Thin

If being overweight is killing tens of millions of Americans because it causes so many deadly diseases, the solution to this crisis seems obvious: Americans who weigh more than is good for them should find a way to weigh less. And indeed that is precisely the message the medical and public health establishment has been broadcasting for decades. The Surgeon General's *Call to Action to Prevent and Decrease Overweight and Obesity*, which assumes an effective strategy for dealing with the health problems associated with overweight is identical to a strategy for making Americans thinner, is merely echoing a century's worth of medical advice. A recent article by Harvard Medical School researchers was even more specific: "Adults should try to maintain a body mass index between 18.5 and 21.9 to minimize their risk of disease" (for an average-height woman, this would mean maintaining a weight between 108 and 127 pounds). And while such an ambitiously restrictive definition of a healthy weight is becoming the medical ideal, even small amounts of weight loss can make a big difference in regard to improved health: According to the NIH, a 10% loss of body mass often leads to significant improvements in blood pressure and glucose tolerance (the latter is critical to avoiding diabetes).

How then are Americans supposed to achieve these goals? Public health authorities assure us the best path to healthy weight loss is a combination of caloric restriction—a.k.a. dieting—and exercise. Unfortunately this classic prescription has an extremely high failure rate: The vast majority of dieters end up regaining all of the weight they lose, and many end up weighing more than they did prior to their attempts to lose weight. Given this record of failure, it's not surprising that the pharmaceutical industry has spent billions of dollars attempting to develop safe and effective weight loss drugs. Although much of the medical and public health establishment is less enthusiastic about the use of diet drugs than it is about dieting per se, many of the most prominent figures in obesity research nevertheless have direct ties to the multibillion-dollar diet drug industry. And for those whom neither dieting nor diet drugs can seem to help, weight loss surgery is becoming an increasingly popular option. After a period of years during which it was frowned upon as a radical and dangerous procedure, gastric bypass surgery has made a big comeback in the course of the last decade: more than one hundred thousand Americans underwent such surgeries in 2003, a figure that has more than tripled in the course of the last five years, and that is expected to continue to skyrocket. (These surgeries remain both highly profitable and extremely dangerous: One in fifty patients dies within a month of undergoing the procedure.)

This, then, is the case against fat: America, we are told, is on the verge of eating itself to death, and therefore the government and private industry must continue to pour resources into the search for a cure to this terrible disease.

Cross-examining the Evidence

According to its advocates, the war on fat is something close to a battle for national survival (this is just one of the many parallels between it and the war on drugs). Ultimately, whether that war is worth the cost requires a close look at the actual evidence. In what follows, I will examine that evidence piece by piece. Readers can decide for themselves how well the case against fat holds together.

Insurance Charts and BMI Tables

If the central claim in the case against fat is that being "overweight" seriously endangers one's health, the core belief of those prosecuting this case is that the BMI tables testify to a strong, predictable relationship between increasing weight and increasing mortality. That, after all, is what most people who ever consider the issue assume when they read that medical and public health authorities have determined a BMI of 25 or above is hazardous to a person's health. This belief, however, is not supported by the available evidence.

In recent years, public health officials have attempted to popularize the BMI tables, partly in response to decades of criticism of the life insurance industry's height-weight charts. As many critics have pointed out, the data from these charts was assembled in a highly unscientific fashion: For example, policyholders reported their own weight (a notoriously unreliable way to collect data), and did so only once—at the time they bought insurance. Furthermore, the charts themselves never did end up correlating with any reliably predictive information about future health prospects. As University of Virginia professor Glenn Gaesser points out, there were many instances in which the MetLife tables labeled people "overweight" whom the actuarial data on which the tables were supposedly based indicated had the lowest mortality risk for their particular cohort. This helps explain why the tables often changed their recommendations, by adding, for example, different body "frames" to their analysis, even though no scientific basis existed—or exists today—for the idea that people fall into groups of well-defined body frames. Indeed, when MetLife issued its most recent version of the tables (in 1983), the company admitted that "[the weights recommended by the tables] are not the weights that minimize illness or the incidence of disease. These weights are not used for underwriting or in the computation of premiums." Yet despite the fact that MetLife does not even use its own tables to price insurance, and that scientists such as Gaesser have demonstrated in detail why these tables are, in his words, "arbitrary, random and meaningless," anti-fat warriors still cite the insurance charts as proof for the claim that fat kills.

What Do Epidemiological Studies
Actually Indicate?

The public health establishment's BMI tables were supposed to replace the haphazard structure of the MetLife charts with a new scientific rigor, as the tables derived their data from large-scale epidemiological studies rather than insurance application forms. But this new rigor soon presented obesity researchers with a problem: Time after time, these studies failed to find the "right" correlations between increasing weight and increasing mortality. For example, here are some figures from what—at the time it was compiled—was the world's largest epidemiological study to date. This study, conducted in Norway in the mid-1980s, followed 1.8 million people for ten years. Consider the following data in light of the government's and the medical establishment's claims that a BMI of 18.5 to 24.9 is optimal, and that people with BMI figures of 25 and above are running major health risks. The *highest* life expectancy (79.7 years) was found among people with BMI figures between 26 and 28, all of whom were overweight according to current U.S. government guidelines. The *lowest* life expectancy (74.2 years) was found among those with BMI figures below 18 (a woman of average height who is 5 pounds below what the government claims is her "optimal" BMI will fall into this highest risk category). Those with BMI figures between 18 and 20—most of whom were at what our public health authorities claim is an optimal weight—had a lower life expectancy than those with BMI figures between 34 and 36: people who according to these same authorities were roughly 60 to 75 pounds "overweight," and therefore seriously "obese."

This study is not unusual. In the late 1980s, obesity researchers Paul Ernsberger and Paul Haskew undertook a comprehensive review of the available epidemiological evidence regarding the relationship between weight and mortality, and concluded that "many studies show that maximum longevity is associated with above average weight." Ernsberger and Haskew pointed out that, contrary to the conventional medical wisdom, increasing body mass did not correlate well with increased risk, and that indeed the correlation sometimes ran in the other direction:

> In a series of eleven prospective studies presented by the International Collaborative Group, not one showed a positive correlation between obesity and mortality by multivariate analysis. On the contrary, three of them found a significant linear decrease in death rate with increasing body weight. In a review of sixteen controlled studies relating body weight and mortality, Reubin Andres stated: "It is concluded that the major population studies of obesity and mortality fail to show that overall obesity leads to greater risk. It is suggested that not only does advice on the subject of obesity need reappraisal but research into possible associated benefits of moderate obesity would be worthwhile." In the seven years since Andres made this statement, more studies have shown the benefits of being heavy.

In the years since Ernsberger, Haskew, and Andres analyzed the available data, other comprehensive surveys have further supported their findings. A particularly compelling illustration of this point is provided by a 1996 study undertaken by scientists at the National Center for Health Statistics and Cornell University. This project analyzed the data from dozens of previous studies, involving a total of more than six hundred thousand subjects with up to a thirty-year follow-up, making it, in the words of one prominent obesity researcher, "one of the most comprehensive analyses of the relationship between mortality and body weight published to date." The results of this analysis should startle anyone who has assumed the government's BMI recommendations are actually justified by the available evidence. Among non-smoking white men the lowest mortality rate was found among those with a BMI between 23 and 29, which means that a large majority of the men who lived longest were "overweight" according to government guidelines. The mortality rate for white men in the supposedly ideal range of 19 to 21 was the same as that for those in the 29 to 31 range (most of whom would be defined currently as "obese"). The researchers were sufficiently struck by this to point out that since their analysis of existing studies had found "increased mortality at moderately low BMI for white men comparable to that found at extreme overweight, which does not appear to be due to smoking or existing disease," it followed that "attention to the health risks of underweight is needed, and body weight recommendations for optimum longevity need to be considered in light of these risks." In regard to non-smoking white women, the study's conclusions were even more striking: The authors concluded the available data indicated that, for such women, the BMI range correlating with the lowest mortality rate was extremely broad, from around 18 to 32, meaning a woman of average height could weigh anywhere within an 80-pound range without seeing any statistically significant change in her risk of premature death.

Again and again, analyses of large-scale epidemiological studies have confirmed this general pattern. For instance, the Pooling Project, which combined the actuarial data from five large American studies, also found the highest mortality in the thinnest cohort. What is most striking about these figures is that the thinnest cohort in this analysis included everyone who weighed less—even just a few pounds less—than the midpoint of the "medium frame desirable weight" figures from the MetLife tables. At the other end of the spectrum the mortality rate in the fattest cohort—those whose weight was more than 40% above the MetLife definitions of desirable weight—was also elevated, but was still lower than that of those in the thin cohort. Between these categories mortality rates bounced around quite a bit, but the combined data in this survey suggested that a weight approximately 25 to 35% *above* the insurance table recommendations was optimal.

Another compelling example is provided by the First National Health and Nutrition Examination Survey (NHANES I), which has followed a large cohort of black and white Americans since 1982. In 1998, results from this survey found that, among black men and women, the lowest mortality rate occurred at a BMI of 27, that is, "overweight." Although among whites the lowest mortality rate was observed at between 24 and 25 (the very top of the government's recommended weight range), the data once again confirmed a broad range of about nine BMI units, between BMI 22 and 31 for blacks, and 20 and 29 for whites, across which there was no significant variation in risk according to BMI (these ranges include about 70% of the U.S. adult population). The authors concluded that their findings "demonstrate a wide range of BMIs consistent with minimum mortality and do not suggest that the optimal BMI is at the lower end of the distribution for any age group."

Yet another recent example comes from the famous Seven Countries Study, which has tracked thousands of men from seven different nations (the United States, Japan, Finland, Italy, Greece, the Netherlands, and the former Yugoslavia) for more than forty years. None of the many medical articles published on the basis of the data from this study have indicated that, in terms of life expectancy, it is better to be thinner than average. Indeed, a recent report on nearly eight thousand Europeans from the study found that thin men (those with a BMI of less than 18.5) had roughly twice the mortality rate of either normal weight or "overweight" men. And this remained true without regard to smoking status. Being "overweight" (BMI 25 to 29.9) had no impact on mortality. Although being "obese" (BMI 30+) did increase mortality, the death rate of men in this category was still lower than that among thin men.

These various examples comprise a small but representative piece of a medical literature that exhibits a strong and consistent pattern. In almost all large-scale epidemiological studies little or no correlation between weight and health can be found for a large majority of the population—and indeed what correlation does exist suggests that it is more dangerous to be just a few pounds "underweight" than dozens of pounds "overweight."

Given this, how are we to make sense of studies whose authors claim provide evidence for what Professors Willett and Stampfer characterize as "a strong international consensus among scientists that overweight (BMI over 25) and obesity are major contributors" to early death? Let us look at four of the most cited studies for the proposition that "overweight" is a deadly epidemic in America today. Each of these studies has generated a great deal of publicity, and has been cited repeatedly by those who are most committed to prosecuting the case against fat. In other words, if fat kills, the most unimpeachable evidence for that proposition should be found within articles such as "Body Weight and Mortality Among Women," "Annual Deaths Attributable to Obesity in the United States," "Years of Life Lost to Obesity," and "Overweight, Obesity and Mortality from Cancer."

Anyone who bothers to examine the evidence in the case against fat with a critical eye will be struck by the radical disconnect between the data in these studies and the conclusions their authors reach. This is actually a common occurrence in the world of obesity research. Glenn Gaesser often performs a thought experiment on his physiology students at the University of Virginia: "I routinely take published papers and cut out everything but the methods and results, and have the students write a title, abstract, introduction, and discussion. You would be surprised at how differently the papers come out." Let us perform a similar experiment on the data from these four articles, which supposedly provide compelling evidence for the proposition that "excess" weight is a deadly health hazard.

Since its 1995 publication in the *New England Journal of Medicine*, "Body Weight and Mortality Among Women" has become the single most cited medical study for the proposition that even small amounts of "overweight" pose a grave health risk. As one of its authors declared at the time of its publication, "We can no longer afford to be complacent about the epidemic of obesity in America. Even mild to moderate overweight is associated with a substantial increase in risk of premature death." Let us look closely at the data from this article, which followed 115,195 nurses for sixteen years. The first point to note is that, relatively speaking, not many women died over the course of the study—4,726, or about 4.5% of the cohort. As several critics subsequently pointed out, the safest generalizations one could draw from the study were that middle-aged, middle-class, white (98% of the cohort) American women have quite low overall mortality rates, and that smoking is a serious health hazard (the death rate among smokers was several times higher than that among non-smokers). Furthermore, the thinnest women in the study were nearly twice as likely to smoke as the fattest women. Given that many women smoke to remain thin, the authors could easily have reached the conclusion that being or remaining thin was the most significant risk factor for the behavior—smoking—that itself was by far the deadliest risk factor in their study. Yet they were not inclined to interpret their data in this fashion.

As for the connection between body mass and mortality, there was little or no risk of increased mortality associated with body mass among the 82% of women in the survey who had BMI figures between, on the one hand, the supposedly ideal range of 19 to 24.9, and, on the other, the supposedly "overweight" range of 25 to 31.9 (this latter group included all the women the study categorized as mildly to moderately obese). Indeed, the comparative mortality between these two groups was nearly identical.

The most remarkable feature of the study's data, in light of the authors' oft-cited claim that their study demonstrated how even mild levels of "overweight" carry significant health risks, is that—if one ignores manipulations of their data that obscured the fact—the women in the study with the lowest mortality rates were found between the 73rd and 84th percentile of body mass. In other words, the women with the lowest death risk were a good deal heavier than average: Indeed, only about one in every six women in the study was heavier than the women in this lowest-risk group. These women, who had BMI figures between 25 and 26.9, would be categorized as overweight by current U.S. government guidelines—guidelines that were lowered to include such women after obesity researchers advocated lowering them in the wake of the conclusions the Nurses' Health Study had reached, despite the fact that the study's data indicated such women had *lower* mortality rates than anyone else! (The article's final sentence is, "The increasingly permissive U.S. weight guidelines may therefore be unjustified and potentially harmful.")

Given all this, how were the authors able to reach their celebrated conclusion that mild to moderate obesity was a substantial health risk? They did so in two ways: by removing smoking from the equation, in order to compare thin non-smoking women to fatter non-smoking women, and by exaggerating the meaning of the data this questionable tactic produced. First, note that in this sort of interpretive context removing smoking from the equation is tantamount to removing anorexia and bulimia from a study that is supposed to measure the relative health risks of fatness and thinness (as mentioned above, smoking is a common weight loss and weight maintenance strategy; and indeed the thin women in the study were far more likely to smoke). Furthermore, even after manipulating their data in this fashion, the authors were able to show only that mildly to moderately obese (non-smoking) women had a negligibly higher mortality risk than (non-smoking) thinner women.

A classic strategy for making small risks seem larger than they are is to note elevations in very small risks, and then to argue as if the impressive relative percentage of increased risk that such elevations often generate is in and of itself something to be alarmed by, even if the overall percentage of risk remains tiny. For example, suppose that Group A consists of twenty-five hundred subjects, and that over the course of a decade five of these people die from cardiovascular disease. Now suppose that Group B consists of four thousand subjects, and that five of the members of this group also die from cardiovascular disease over the same ten-year span. One way of characterizing these figures is to note that people in Group A were 60% more likely to die of cardiovascular disease than people in Group B. One could even choose to call this "a substantial increase in risk of premature death." But in point of fact the risk of dying from cardiovascular disease for people in *either* group was tiny. That, one would think, would be the most salient point when attempting to assess the various health risks these people faced.

Consider in this regard the authors' claim that mild obesity increased the mortality risk associated with it by 60%. The authors focused on cardiovascular disease among non-smoking women, because this portion of their data appeared to demonstrate the closest link between mortality and an obesity-associated condition. But even this conclusion was problematic. Only a miniscule percentage of non-smoking women—184—died of cardiovascular disease over the sixteen-year course of the study (this figure represents fewer than one out of every six hundred women in the study as a whole). In particular, very few women with a BMI under 29 were in this category. Yet the press release accompanying the study emphasized that such "mildly" obese women had a 60% greater mortality rate than thinner women, primarily as a result of elevated rates of cardiovascular disease. Although literally true, this was quite misleading. Since the death rate among thin (non-smoking) women was so low, a 60% increase over that rate still constituted a negligible risk. In other words, 60% more than almost nothing is still almost nothing. What this study actually demonstrated was that the odds that a mildly "obese" middle-aged middle-class non-smoking white woman would die of cardiovascular disease (or anything else) over the sixteen-year course of the study were extremely low. That they were slightly lower for a thinner woman with the same background does not alter that fundamental fact. And again, even this modest increase in mortality risk was produced only after removing smoking from the equation.

I have focused at length on the Nurses' Health Study article, both because it has received so much publicity, and because the disconnect between its data and its conclusions is quite typical of what one finds when one looks more closely at the epidemiological studies that supposedly prove the case against fat. Similar criticisms can be made of "Annual Deaths Attributable to Obesity," "Years of Life Lost to Obesity," and "Overweight, Obesity and Mortality from Cancer." Rather than going into as much detail in regard to these articles, I will merely point to some striking features in their data, confirming the same general point.

"Annual Deaths Attributable to Obesity in the United States," which appeared in the *Journal of the American Medical Association* (*JAMA*) in 1999, is the source for the endlessly repeated statistic that overweight causes around three hundred thousand extra deaths in the United States every year. (This "fact" has been cited in the major media more than seventeen hundred times in the last two years alone.) Yet even before basic methodological questions are raised about surveys of this type (see the next section), we should note that, once again, this survey reveals a very broad, U-shaped risk curve. For example, the study's data indicate that persons with a BMI of 20 run the same risk of premature death as those with BMIs of 30, even though the former are "ideally" thin, while the latter are "obese." And both these groups have a slightly higher risk than persons at a BMI of 25 ("overweight"). One would never guess from the authors' discussion of their findings, and the conclusions they reach, that their data actually showed little or no fluctuation in risk associated with differing body mass for the large majority of the people included in their study.

Furthermore, as Glenn Gaesser points out, studies have consistently failed to find any correlation between increasing BMI and higher mortality in people sixty-five and over, and 78% of the approximately 2.3 million annual deaths in the United States occur among people who are at least sixty-five. Thus 78% of all deaths lack even the beginning of a statistical link with BMI. "That leaves," Gaesser told me, "five hundred thousand annual deaths in persons under sixty-five that *might* be related to BMI. These include deaths from every possible cause: motor vehicle and other accidents, homicides, suicides, cigarettes, alcohol, microbial agents, toxic agents, drug abuse, etc., etc. To think that 60% (i.e., three hundred thousand) of these deaths are due to body fat is absolutely preposterous."

"Years of Life Lost Due to Obesity" appeared in *JAMA* in January of 2003. It, like its 1999 predecessor in the same journal, was immediately seized upon by the weight loss industry as proof of the devastating health effects caused by above-average weight. It, too, received widespread coverage in the mass media. Yet the authors' conclusion that "obesity appears to lessen life expectancy markedly, especially among younger adults," is, to say the least, a controversial interpretation of their data. For example, among African Americans, the authors' data indicate that the entire "overweight" range of BMI 25 to 29.9 is actually optimal, and that, in their own words, "the pattern among black men and women suggests that the only category in which the relative mortality rate is consistently and substantially elevated is among black women with BMIs of less than 18.5." Indeed, among black women no elevated mortality associated with increasing weight was observed at all until a BMI of 37 (for an average-height woman, this would be 223 pounds). Among whites, elevations in mortality rates were negligible until BMIs in the mid-30s, and even then most of the increased risk was seen among people who had gotten extraordinarily fat at a young age. Yet what the authors emphasized, and what the media reported, was that portion of their data indicating things such as that a twenty-year-old white man with a BMI of over 45 (i.e., someone who weighs more than 315 pounds at this age) will on average lose thirteen years of life expectancy in comparison to an "ideal" weight individual of the same age. While this is an interesting piece of information, emphasizing it obscures the fact that such people are very rare, and that, again, for the vast majority of people classified by the government as overweight or obese, the study found little or no increased risk associated with increasing body mass.

"Overweight, Obesity and Mortality from Cancer," published in the *New England Journal of Medicine* in April of 2003, was the subject of front-page stories in many of the nation's leading newspapers. For example, a *Los Angeles Times* article reported that the study provided "the first definitive account of the relationship between obesity and cancer." The article went on to quote the study's authors to the effect that perhaps as many as ninety thousand deaths per year from cancer could be avoided if all adults maintained a BMI below 25 throughout their lives. The disjunction between this study's actual data and the alarmist headlines its authors helped generate is especially remarkable. Among supposedly "ideal weight" individuals (BMI 18.5 to 24.9), the study observed a mortality rate from cancer of 4.5 deaths per one thousand subjects. Among "overweight" individuals (BMI 25 to 29.9—a category that currently includes about twice as many adult Americans as the "ideal weight" cohort), the cancer mortality rate was 4.4 deaths per one thousand subjects. In other words, "overweight" people actually had a *lower* overall cancer mortality rate than "ideal weight" individuals! Among the "moderately obese"—people weighing anywhere from about

35 to 70 pounds more than the government's recommended maximum—
the death rate was 5.1 per one thousand subjects. That is, even among
people who would be considered quite fat, the correlation between increasing weight and cancer mortality yielded a total of approximately
one extra cancer death among every two thousand such people in the
study. Among people weighing 75 to 100 pounds more than the recommended maximum, the death rate was 5.8 per one thousand (i.e.,
slightly more than one extra cancer death per every one thousand such
people). And among the extraordinarily fat—people weighing, on average, much more than 100 pounds over the recommended maximum—
the death rate was 6.8 cancer deaths per one thousand subjects.

In short, this study actually found a *negative* correlation between
increasing weight and cancer mortality for the majority of the 135 million Americans who are currently characterized as overweight and
obese, and only a miniscule increase in risk among even extremely fat
people. (Consider what it says about the pervasiveness of America's
weight hysteria that the "morbidly obese" women in this study were
less likely to die of cancer than the "ideal weight" men. It seems unlikely that this typical statistic—in developed nations, "morbidly obese"
women routinely have longer life expectancies than "ideal weight"
men—will lead to a Surgeon General's Call to Action to Prevent and
Decrease Masculinity.)

Despite their authors' claims, the data from these four studies,
which represent the core of the prosecution's case against fat, actually
ends up reflecting what the epidemiological literature in general suggests. While very fat and very thin people tend to die sooner than average, there appears to be a broad range of weight—running roughly
from a BMI in the high teens to one somewhere well into the thirties—
at which little or no correlation between weight and early mortality
can be found (this range includes most of the people the government
now classifies as "overweight" and "obese"). Indeed many such studies
find the lowest mortality levels at BMI figures that are currently classified as "overweight." Furthermore, given current government guidelines, it appears that the average person is better off being 50 or even
75 pounds "overweight" than 5 pounds "underweight." The bottom
line is that anyone who examines the actual epidemiological data will
discover this devastating flaw at the heart of the prosecution's case
against fat. And this flaw has been exposed even *before* the defense has

presented its strongest arguments: arguments that will begin by pointing out the severe weaknesses that plague epidemiological analyses of
this sort.

Does Fat Really Cause Disease?

As we have seen, the first major premise of the case against fat—
that being of more than average weight is a major contributor to early
mortality—is largely unsupported by the epidemiological evidence.
What about the second premise—that, in the words of the public
health establishment, being "overweight" puts a person "at risk for developing many diseases, especially heart disease, diabetes and cancer?" As we are about to see, this claim is highly misleading in two
quite different ways. First, when anti-fat warriors discuss correlations
between increasing body mass and various diseases, they invariably
leave out the other half of the story: specifically the part that chronicles both the ambiguity of the evidence in regard to the positive correlations between fat and disease, and the many *negative* correlations
between increasing weight and serious illness. Second, such arguments either ignore or gloss over the great difficulties that arise when
one attempts to establish a causal, rather than a merely correlative, relationship between body mass and disease.

Let's begin by looking at the three major diseases that are most
often mentioned by those prosecuting the case against fat: heart disease, diabetes, and cancer.

Heart Disease

Most Americans, and indeed most doctors, simply assume that the
heavier you are, the more likely it is you will suffer from coronary
artery disease—hence the various clichés about "artery-clogging" fast
food and the like. Yet several studies have specifically investigated the
question of whether a high percentage of body fat correlates with the
incidence of coronary artery disease. Answer: No, it does not. Even
massively obese men and women do not appear to be more prone to
vascular disease than average. It has been estimated that somewhere
between 1 and 5 percent of the change in risk for heart disease across
populations can be attributed to increasing body mass—yet such increases are cited routinely as "critical" factors in heightening one's risk

for the disease. Indeed, as we shall see, there is a great deal of evidence that weight *loss* increases the risk for cardiovascular disease among "overweight" individuals, and some studies suggest that obesity actually protects against vascular disease.

It is true that increasing weight is associated with high blood pressure and certain types of heart disease. But even here there is considerable evidence that this correlation is not necessarily a product of being fat, but rather of losing and then regaining weight. Obese patients who have been put on very low-calorie diets subsequently display much higher rates of congestive heart failure (the form of heart disease most closely associated with obesity) than equally fat people who did not attempt to lose weight in the first place. Similar effects have been noted in nonexperimental settings. For example, when the siege of Leningrad was lifted during World War II, hospitalizations for hypertension increased by 50%, as people who had been starving regained weight lost during the siege. Furthermore, among those who suffer from hypertension the mortality rate from the disease is two to three times lower among heavy individuals as compared to thin persons—and yet "overweight" hypertensives are advised routinely to treat their condition through weight loss. Glenn Gaesser points out the potentially deadly irony: "If a hypertensive obese person follows the advice to lose weight in order to lower blood pressure and the remedy doesn't work [as it often doesn't], then what you have is a weight-reduced hypertensive who is now statistically more likely to die from cardiovascular disease than before . . . this may help explain [why] men and women who have undergone sustained weight loss are at a greater risk of cardiovascular disease mortality."

The biggest evidentiary problem for those who insist there is a strong causal link between increasing weight and heart disease is that deaths from heart disease have been plunging at precisely the same time that obesity rates have been skyrocketing. The death rate from heart disease and hypertension is less than half of what it was a generation ago: Indeed, NIH statisticians calculate that if the death rate had remained what it was in 1970, 1.1 million more Americans per year would be dying of these diseases (over this same time frame, obesity rates have more than doubled). And those who do die of heart disease are much older: A generation ago, the stereotypical victim of heart disease was a man in his fifties who suddenly dropped dead. Today, "that death rate is so low that we're no longer able to track it," says Dr.

Teri Manolio of the National Heart, Lung and Blood Institute. And, notes the *New York Times*, "despite the obesity epidemic, these trends are continuing with no end in sight." That obesity may in the end have little to do with heart disease is apparently too simple a hypothesis to commend itself to those who compile and report on these statistics.

Diabetes

Indictments in the case against fat invariably focus on diabetes, because Type 2 diabetes is much more common among heavier-than-average people. It has become routine to claim that America is about to be overwhelmed by a diabetes epidemic, that for the first time Type 2 diabetes is being seen among children, etc., and that the solution to this crisis is to make fat people thin. The facts, however, are considerably more complicated than these claims acknowledge. Paul Ernsberger, a professor at the Case Western Reserve University School of Medicine who has studied both obesity and the medical literature regarding it for more than twenty years, questions every aspect of the conventional story. "Actually," he points out, "there is no hard data that says blood sugar levels are rising. Instead, there are many reports of telephone surveys where people are asked if they have diabetes. Diabetes used to be tremendously under-diagnosed—less than one-third of diabetics were aware they had the disease." This has changed, says Ernsberger, because of aggressive educational programs designed to encourage more testing, and mass screenings of millions of Americans for the disease. "Also," he notes, "the definition of diabetes was changed from a fasting blood sugar of 140 to a blood sugar of 126. Thus, millions of Americans became diabetic overnight. We are also an aging population, and diabetes incidence rises exponentially after age fifty. There is also considerable confusion—many doctors are telling people they are 'borderline diabetic,' or to watch out for diabetes, or to lose weight to prevent diabetes, and patients will misunderstand and think they are already diabetic."

Ernsberger sees much of this as good news, "because far fewer people are going undiagnosed. Treatments for Type 2 diabetes have improved tremendously, and most cases can be controlled through a combination of pills, healthier diet and regular exercise. So far, there is no evidence that fasting blood sugar levels have increased in the population." As for claims that we are for the first time seeing Type 2 diabetes among children, and especially inner-city minority children,

Ernsberger points out that childhood Type 2 diabetes "has been known for decades, but no one ever determined its prevalence until recently. Until recently, epidemiological studies focused on white sub-urban middle-aged men and women, while children, minorities and inner-city residents were ignored." Indeed, even as organizations such as the Centers for Disease Control have issued warnings about a sup-posed epidemic of Type 2 diabetes, their own statistics indicate that rates of the disease hardly altered over the last decade, despite the obesity "epidemic." (According to the CDC, over the course of the 1990s the incidence of Type 2 diabetes increased from 8.2 to 8.6 per-cent, while the obesity rate rose by 61%.)

Furthermore, as we shall see, several recent studies indicate that the key to avoiding Type 2 diabetes is not to try to lose weight (indeed there is much evidence that dieters are far more prone to the dis-ease than average), but rather to make lifestyle changes in regard to activity levels and dietary content that greatly reduce the risk of con-tracting the disease, whether or not such changes lead to any weight loss.

Cancer

In February of 2003, the American Cancer Society announced plans to hold a "Great American Weigh In," modeled on the Great American Smokeout, the Society's thirty-year-old effort to encourage people to give up smoking. "One-third of cancer deaths are related to diet and inactivity," said the group's director of nutrition and physical activity, Colleen Doyle. She claimed that about 186,000 lives per year could be saved by changing peoples' living habits. Note that it is typi-cal of those prosecuting the case against fat that they fail to notice the facts they cite do not actually involve any claims about weight per se. If people are getting cancer because they are too sedentary and be-cause they eat unhealthy foods, it does not follow that it's necessary or even desirable for them to lose weight, as long as they become more active and eat a healthier diet. But do people of more-than-average weight actually face a greater risk of dying from cancer? Here again, the medical literature tells a very different story from that related by our anti-fat warriors.

Over the past three decades, according to Glenn Gaesser's survey of the literature, between thirty-five and forty medical studies have found increasing body mass to be associated with a lower incidence of various cancers, and with lower mortality from cancer. At least nine separate studies have found an association between increasing weight and a lower overall mortality from cancer of all types. Indeed, Paul Ernsberger notes that total cancer death rates fall with rising BMI in almost every study he has seen. For example, the landmark Seven Countries Study, which has followed nearly thirteen thousand men from around the world for more than forty years, has to this point observed that the risk of dying from cancer decreases with increasing relative weight. To quote from the study itself, "Relative body weight (body mass index) was an important negative risk factor, meaning that the risk of dying from cancer decreased with increasing relative weight." Other studies have shown that heavier people are less prone to suffer from stomach cancer, lung cancer, premenopausal breast cancer (which is far deadlier than postmenopausal breast cancer; furthermore, the association between thinness and premenopausal breast cancer is stronger than that between fatness and postmenopausal breast cancer), and meningioma. The association between less-than-average weight and higher overall cancer mortality remains even when studies control for smoking, and for "occult wasting" (i.e., weight loss brought on by a preexisting disease). And even those studies that suggest a link between increasing weight and cancer risk, such as the April 2003 *New England Journal of Medicine* article discussed above, tend to produce quite ambiguous data (recall that this study found the lowest cancer risk among the "overweight," and only a slightly elevated cancer risk among all but the very fattest subjects).

Does Fat Protect Against Disease?

The oft-noted association between increasing weight and decreasing cancer risk is just one example out of many similar such relationships. Diseases and syndromes that various medical studies indicate are less common among heavier people include emphysema, chronic obstructive pulmonary disease, hip fracture, vertebral fracture, tuberculosis, anemia, peptic ulcer, and chronic bronchitis, among others. Indeed, how many people are aware that heavier women have much lower rates of osteoporosis, which is a very common and serious condition among older women? (There is considerable evidence that chronic dieting causes loss of bone mass, which greatly increases the risk of developing osteoporosis.) These are not rare or insignificant diseases. Consider the potential implications for public health of the fact that hip fractures are two and a half times less likely to occur among heavier women. Hip fracture is a leading cause of both death and permanent disability among older women (in Great Britain more women die from osteoporosis-related hip fracture than from breast, cervical, and uterine cancer combined).

In short, the charge that being fat causes deadly diseases is both simplistic and one-sided. The positive correlations between increasing weight and conditions such as heart disease and diabetes are much more problematic than the standard anti-fat story admits; furthermore, there are many negative correlations between increasing weight and various common and extremely serious diseases. If we were to employ the logic of the anti-fat warriors, does this latter fact mean that Americans should be encouraged to *gain* weight so as to protect themselves from, among other things, cancer, osteoporosis, and most of the major pulmonary diseases? This question raises an issue we have not yet touched on—one that has profound implications for the case against fat.

Is Getting Thin the Answer?

To this point we have focused on the epidemiological evidence, without taking into account the serious limitations of epidemiology. The most serious of these is that observational studies—that is, studies that follow a pool of subjects for a number of years in order to observe correlations between various risk factors and disease—cannot by themselves prove causation. Of course some correlations are so striking that they create a strong prima facie case for a causal relationship. For example, the fact that heavy smokers are 3,000 percent more likely to develop lung cancer than non-smokers by itself provides compelling evidence of a causal link between smoking and lung cancer. Studies observe about fifty more deaths per year from lung cancer among every ten thousand heavy smokers, as compared to every ten thousand non-smokers. By contrast, an "overweight" woman faces a 13% increased risk for postmenopausal breast cancer, meaning that studies observe about *one* extra postmenopausal breast cancer death per year among every ten thousand overweight women. Epidemiologists usually ignore associations of this magnitude, since they could easily be accounted for by any of a host of other variables. Yet in the context of weight, even the weakest associations are routinely treated as if they were equivalent to the sort of association seen between smoking and lung cancer.

In general, how meaningful are the associations between weight and health? Although we have seen that most groups of people whom the government and the health establishment label "overweight" and "obese" do not, on average, suffer from worse health or shorter life expectancy than so-called ideal weight individuals, there are some groups of heavier individuals—usually those with BMI figures in the mid-30s and above—who do. Yet this fact by itself does not prove either that such people's health problems are caused by their excess weight, or that their health would improve if they lost weight. To begin to answer these questions, it is necessary to control for at least some of the many other factors that disproportionately affect the heaviest people in our society, and that also correlate with poor health: most notably sedentary lifestyle, poor diet, dieting-induced weight fluctuation, diet drug use, poverty, access to and discrimination in health care, and social discrimination generally.

In other words, if some fat people are less healthy than average, is this because they are fat, or because they are poor, sedentary, prone to the weight cycling that afflicts dieters, more likely to use dangerous diet drugs, and so forth? Glenn Gaesser points out that more epidemiology is not likely to provide wholly satisfactory answers to these questions, "due," he says, "to the inexactness of epidemiology." A particularly interesting and ironic admission of this point was made by Charles Hennekens, one of the authors of the Nurses' Health Study discussed above. When interviewed for a *New York Times* story exploring the often contradictory advice issuing from the authors of epidemiological studies, Hennekens admitted that, "Epidemiology is a crude and inexact science . . . we tend to overstate findings, either because we want attention or more grant money."

While Dr. Hennekens' candor is refreshing, it represents a significant admission against interest by a key witness in the case against fat. For what we have ignored up to this point is that the entire case against fat hinges not only on the inaccurate assumption that increasing body weight correlates well with ill health and early death, but also on three further assumptions: that heavier people will be healthier if they lose weight; that the health benefits of attempting to lose weight will outweigh the possible risks; and that some reasonably reliable method or methods exist to carry out this prescription. Naturally, such assumptions cannot be supported by epidemiological studies that fail to control for the risk factors that these assumptions implicate. Studies that do not control for factors such as dieting, diet drug use, fitness, activity levels, etc., cannot tell us whether whatever ill health they discover among larger people is due to "excess" weight, or to some combination of these and other factors. *And yet all of the studies that are most often cited by anti-fat warriors almost completely fail to control for such factors.*

When I reviewed the epidemiological evidence earlier in this chapter, I did not mention this enormous hole at the center of the case against fat. I wanted to emphasize that even those studies that are most often cited by anti-fat warriors largely fail to support the conclusions their authors draw from them. This remains true even when we take these studies at face value, that is, even if we assume they control adequately for the most crucial variables when exploring the question of whether fat causes disease and early mortality, or merely serves as a marker for the presence of other factors that are actually responsible for whatever ill health can be found among the heavier than average. But in fact these studies almost never control for any of the variables mentioned above. For example, "Annual Deaths Attributable to Obesity in the United States," the *JAMA* study responsible for the "fact" that fat kills three hundred thousand Americans per year, contains the following remarkable sentence in its statement of methods: "Our calculations assume that all (controlling for age, sex and smoking) excess mortality in obese people is due to their adiposity." The authors of this study did not try to determine the extent to which sedentary lifestyle, dietary content, dieting, diet drugs, poverty, discrimination in health care, and social discrimination in general, among other factors, accounted for some, most, or indeed quite possibly all of the excess mortality they observed among some groups of heavier people. In other words, they created the validity of their conclusion by sheer definition: They "discovered" that all excess mortality among the heavier than average was caused by "excess" weight by simply assuming this was the case!

In this regard, the data from this article are typical of those used in large-scale epidemiological studies. To begin to determine whether whatever excess morbidity and mortality can be observed among some groups of "obese" people is caused by their "excess" weight, it's necessary to look at the medical literature that has explored the effects on health of some of the variables that these studies ignore. Let us focus on three: dieting, diet drugs, and fitness and activity levels.

Dieting

The case against fat proceeds on the assumption that if a fat person becomes thin, that person will acquire the health characteristics of people who were thin in the first place. It also assumes that there is some reasonably safe and reliable method for producing this result. Note that although the first assumption may seem like simple common sense, it is, like many commonsensical assumptions, quite dubious. If a person who is physiologically inclined to be fat loses weight, this does not transform that person into someone who is physiologically inclined to be thin. To understand the implications of this distinction, consider that bald men die sooner, on average, than hirsute men, probably because bald men have higher levels of testosterone, which appear to lower life expectancy. Given this, surely no one would conclude that giving a bald man hair implants would improve his prospects for long life. To test whether turning people who are physiologically inclined to be fat into thin people actually improves their health, or is instead the equivalent of giving bald men hair implants, it would be necessary to take a statistically significant group of fat people, make them thin, and then keep them thin for long enough to see whether or not their overall health then mirrored that of people who were physiologically inclined to be thin. No one has ever successfully conducted such a study, for a very simple reason: No one knows how to turn fat people into thin people.

This statement is in one sense shocking, despite the fact that there are few better-established empirical propositions in the entire field of medicine. How can this be? After all, as those who prosecute the case against fat never cease to remind us, everyone knows how to lose weight: Eat less and exercise more. In theory, this regimen should make people thin. In practice, it does not. For more than a century now, the medical profession has been telling people that to become thin they need to restrict caloric intake (diet) and increase their activity levels. Hundreds of millions of Americans have spent much of their lives trying to follow this advice. One result of this prescription has been that, for many decades, an increasing percentage of the population has become "overweight" and "obese." As William Bennett and Joel Gurin pointed out twenty years ago in their book *The Dieter's Dilemma: Eating Less and Weighing More,* "the standard 'sensible' recommendations to change eating habits and diligently use caloric charts are no more than elaborate folklore, expressions of faith in a world that ought to exist, but in fact does not." More Americans than ever are dieting: On any given day, approximately seventy million adults are dieting to lose weight, and another forty-five million are dieting to maintain their current weight. These percentages tripled over the course of the last generation. And the result? Americans weigh on average 15 pounds more than they did twenty years ago. (The government's own statistics indicate that somewhere between 88 and 93% of all "obese" Americans are dieting. In other words, almost all fat Americans are already undertaking the "cure" that obesity researchers and the weight loss industry recommend for their "disease.")

The vast majority of people who attempt to lose weight eventually gain all the weight they lose back. A significant percentage of them gain back more than they lost: at least a third or so of such people followed for five years or more, according to Paul Ernsberger. One consequence of this fact is that we simply don't know if people who lose a large amount of weight and keep it off permanently improve their health by doing so. This is what we do know: Tens of millions of Americans are trying—more or less constantly—to lose 20 or 30 pounds (25 pounds tends to be the average figure cited in surveys of dieters). If you ask them why most will tell you they are doing so for the sake of their health, often on the advice of their doctors. Yet Glenn Gaesser notes that numerous studies—more than two dozen in the last twenty years alone—have found that weight loss of this magnitude (and indeed of even as little as 10 pounds) leads to an increased risk of premature death, sometimes by an order of several hundred percent. By contrast, during this same time frame only around four studies have found that weight loss leads to lower mortality rates—and one of these found an eleven-hour increase in life expectancy per pound lost (i.e., the equivalent of an extra month of life in return for a permanent 50-pound weight loss).

Initially, studies of the former sort were dismissed by those prosecuting the case against fat: It was claimed such studies failed to control adequately for smoking, or for the effects of preexisting disease. Yet recent studies that controlled carefully for these factors have observed the same effect. For example, in the early 1990s a major American Cancer Society study showed weight loss to be associated with higher mortality, even after screening out smokers and all deaths that took place within a few years of an individual's entry into the study. And a follow-up to this study concluded that healthy "obese" women were better off if they *didn't* lose weight. In this study, healthy women who intentionally lost weight over a period of a year or longer suffered an increased risk of premature death from cancer, cardiovascular disease, and all other causes that was up to 70% higher than that of healthy women who didn't intentionally lose weight (unintentional weight gain among these women had no effect on mortality). A 1999 report based on the same data pool found similar results for men.

The only other large study to look into the question of the health effects of intentional weight loss—the Iowa Women's Health Study— produced some rather extraordinary data in regard to the assumption that trying to get thin is the appropriate "cure" for the "disease" of above-average weight. The Iowa study is particularly striking, in that it featured no less than 108 different statistical comparisons, based on age, initial weight and health status, and cause of death. In seventy-nine of these comparisons, intentional weight loss was associated with higher mortality rates. By contrast, the number of comparisons in which intentional weight loss ended up being associated with lower mortality rates was zero. This is especially significant information, given that the Iowa study is one of only a few studies that have distinguished between intentional and unintentional weight loss when measuring the effects of weight loss on health.

Several other recent studies have found associations between weight loss and an increased risk of death. In Steven Blair's ongoing long-term longitudinal study of the effects of physical fitness on health, involving more than seventy thousand subjects, a weight loss of more than 5% among men with BMI figures of 26 to 29 increased the risk of cardiovascular disease mortality by nearly 200%, as compared to similarly "overweight" men who maintained stable weights. In the ongoing Harvard Alumni Study, the largest amount of weight *gain*, in physically active men, has correlated with the lowest mortality risk. Yet the "get thin to live longer" message being promulgated by those prosecuting the case against fat is so pervasive that it leads to attempts to produce weight loss even among subgroups in which lower BMI and weight loss both correlate especially well with increased mortality and reduced lifespan, most notably older persons.

For example, a recent article in a magazine published by the American Association of Retired Persons advocates weight loss among the elderly, noting that the National Heart, Lung and Blood Institute of the NIH approves of weight loss among people as old as eighty. And some nursing homes are apparently putting residents on restricted-calorie meal plans if their weight is above a BMI of 25. Such recommendations fly in the face of a host of recent studies indicating that weight loss can be especially dangerous for older persons, including those who are "overweight" or "obese." For instance, a 2002 study of a group of men and women who averaged seventy-one years of age found an increased risk of death with a weight loss of 10 pounds or more, even in diabetics. Another 2002 study found that, among the elderly, a BMI under 24 (high end of the supposedly "ideal" range), or any amount of weight loss, were both risks for premature death. The latter finding applied to the "obese" as well as to the thin members of the study. In 2001 a study reported that, among older people, a weight loss of only 5% increased death rate regardless of starting weight, and regardless of the presence of major illness, while weight gain had no effect on mortality. A 2001 study of postmenopausal women who had never smoked found a beneficial effect from weight gain among those with a BMI of 25 or below. And a 2002 metanalysis of thirty-one clinical trials showed conclusively that weight gain in underweight older persons prospectively reduced mortality by about one-third. Commenting on this recent literature, leading obesity researcher Paul Ernsberger notes that "it's interesting that clinical trials of weight loss have never shown a longevity benefit, but several clinical trials of weight *gain* show it to be correlated with improved longevity!"

The reasons why recent weight loss so often correlates with increased mortality risk, even when one controls for smoking and preexisting disease, are not well understood. Nevertheless certain aspects of the medical literature are suggestive, in particular studies that indicate weight cycling (a.k.a. yo-yo dieting) is a major factor in the development of clogged arteries, congestive heart failure, hypertension, and other serious health problems. Indeed, dieters as a group run up to double the risk of developing cardiovascular disease and Type 2 diabetes when compared to "overweight" people who do not diet. This may be a result of the fact that dieting often leads to bingeing, which is extremely unhealthy, since it is driven by cravings for high-fat, high-sugar foods (indeed, the more often a person diets, the stronger these cravings become). These foods, when consumed by people who have been depriving themselves of adequate caloric intake, are quickly metabolized into visceral body fat, which is far more dangerous to health than subcutaneous fat. (Large people who do not diet tend to have high percentages of subcutaneous fat, but low percentages of visceral fat. Also, physical activity burns visceral fat very quickly, which helps explain why, as we shall see, activity levels are far more important to health than weight.)

What about claims that even small amounts of weight loss have beneficial health effects for people suffering from hypertension and Type 2 diabetes? On closer inspection, these claims are based on studies in which sedentary people with poor dietary habits became physically active and began eating a more nutritious diet. Such studies indicate that the health benefits of these sorts of lifestyle changes are almost wholly independent of whether these changes led to any significant weight loss. As Ernsberger notes, statements to the effect that even a 10% weight reduction can be highly beneficial actually "prove that body weight is nearly irrelevant to health. People who weigh 300 pounds and then lose 10% of their body weight on a balanced low-fat diet rich in fruits and vegetables are still 'morbidly obese,' but their blood sugar, blood pressure and cholesterol have all improved." He points out that "physiologically there is little difference between a 270-pound person maintaining a healthy lifestyle and a 110-pound person. How then can we say that body fat is so deadly? Doesn't this prove that it is lifestyle, not body fat, that is crucial?"

The prevalence of—and the devastating health effects that sometimes follow from—yo-yo dieting, along with the high mortality rates found among people who are just a few pounds under what the government and the health establishment have mischaracterized as an "ideal weight," both provide powerful evidence for the proposition that attempting to lose weight causes far more damage to our health than maintaining even very high weight levels. And even if it were true that heavier people would be healthier if they lost weight, this would still be irrelevant for the purposes of public health policy if most people who intentionally lose weight then regain it, as in fact they do. Although we don't actually know if "overweight" people would be healthier if they lost weight and kept it off (the evidence reviewed above suggests they would not), it has become clear that the vast majority of people who lose weight soon regain it, and often more, and that this sort of weight cycling is hazardous to their health. As Glenn Gaesser has pointed out, given what we know about relative rates of dangerous weight loss practices across different weight groups, studies that purport to show a link between higher mortality and higher BMI are more logically interpreted as indicating a direct relationship between higher mortality and higher rates of dieting and diet drug use. Under these circumstances, advising "overweight" people to lose weight is tantamount to prescribing a drug that causes the disease it is supposed to cure.

Diet Drugs

Given that the medical establishment's traditional "cure" for the "disease" of being heavier than average (advising people to eat less and exercise more) appears to have ended up making Americans a good deal fatter than they would be otherwise, it's not surprising that pharmacology has attempted to succeed where dieting alone has failed. And, despite the often severe side effects associated with their use, drugs remain the staple of the diet trade. Indeed, the search for a magic bullet that can be sold to tens of millions of Americans desperate to conform to unrealistic and potentially dangerous body ideals has become a kind of Grail-like quest for the American pharmaceutical industry.

The list of side effects from the most popular diet drugs is long: Accelerated heart rate, increased blood pressure, palpitations, dry mouth, blurred vision, and light-headedness are among the most common. Long-term use has led to damaged heart muscle, kidney failure, pulmonary hypertension, and stroke.

A new Yale University study indicates that women between the ages of eighteen and forty-nine who have used appetite suppressants containing phenylpropanolamine face an increased risk for hemorrhagic stroke of 1,558% (this over-the-counter drug was being used by approximately nine million Americans at any given time during the late 1990s). This is just one of several common appetite suppressants that have been implicated in numerous fatalities. For example, recently four prominent athletes—football players Kory Stringer, Rashidi Wheeler, and Devaughn Darling, along with major league pitcher Steve Bechler—have collapsed during workouts and died after using diet drugs containing ephedra, a cheap (anyone with twenty dollars to spare can purchase over one hundred doses) over-the-counter herbal stimulant known among college students as "legal speed."

Tellingly, despite our otherwise heavily regulated and criminalized pharmacological culture, diet drugs often end up facing more relaxed regulatory hurdles than drugs designed to fight diseases such as cancer and AIDS. In her book *Dispensing with the Truth: The Victims, the Drug Companies, and the Dramatic Story Behind the Battle over Fen-phen*, Alicia Mundy chronicles how the bureaucratic struggle surrounding the FDA approval and subsequent recall of dexfenfluramine (Redux) and its pharmacological cousin fen-phen provides a classic cautionary tale of how America's obsession with weight loss can intensify the phenomenon of regulatory capture. ("Regulatory capture" is a term used by administrative law scholars to describe how regulated industries often end up controlling the administrative agencies that are responsible for minimizing the socially destructive side effects of the desire for a fat bottom line.) Given that dexfenfluramine has since been associated with various fatal conditions, thus leading to billions of dollars of legal liability for its makers, the fanaticism with which certain prominent obesity researchers· sought its approval has in retrospect taken on a grimly humorous tinge. (After the FDA hearing at which its approval was temporarily blocked, noted anti-fat warrior Dr. Judith Stern opined that any panelists who opposed the drug's approval "ought to be shot.")

Fitness and Activity Levels

Over the past twenty years, scientists have gathered a wealth of evidence indicating that cardiovascular and metabolic fitness, and the activity levels that promote such fitness, are far more important predictors of both overall health and mortality risk than weight. Yet none of the studies most often cited for the proposition that fat kills makes any serious attempt to control for these variables. And indeed, when studies of this type do claim to make such attempts, the methodology employed can be almost farcical. For example, a highly publicized study authored by June Stevens and others, which appeared in the *New England Journal of Medicine* in 1998, and which purported to control for activity levels, did so by asking subjects the following question once, at the time of their entry into the study: "How much exercise do you get (work or play): None, slight, moderate, or heavy?" (Self-assessments of this type have been shown to be almost completely unreliable.)

Rather than pretending that such inadequate methods can provide us with reliable knowledge, let us look at studies that have made a serious attempt to measure the effects of fitness and activity levels on health, especially as these factors relate to body mass. The most extensive work of this sort has been carried out by Steven Blair and his colleagues at Dallas' Cooper Institute. The institute's Aerobics Center Longitudinal Study has, over the course of the past two decades, compiled an extensive database that tracks the health, weight, and basic fitness levels of more than seventy thousand people. Unlike traditional studies of the effect of weight on health—which as we have seen either ignore the role played by fitness and activity levels, or merely ask participants to decide for themselves if they are active or not—the Aerobics Center's study gives regular treadmill stress tests to its participants. This has allowed its researchers to track with great precision the relationship over time between weight, fitness levels, and health. What Blair and his colleagues have discovered is that, quite simply, when researchers take into account the activity levels and resulting fitness of the people being studied, body mass appears to have no relevance to health whatsoever. In Blair's studies obese people—not merely the "overweight," but people with BMI figures of 30 and higher—who engage in at least moderate levels of physical activity have around one half the mortality rate of sedentary people who maintain supposedly ideal weight levels. This remains true whether the heavier people have high or low percentages of body fat. Moreover, the overall health and mortality rates of heavy active people are identical with those of "ideal weight" people who also engage in at least moderate levels of physical activity.

For example, a Cooper Institute study published in the *Journal of the American Medical Association* involving thirteen thousand subjects indicated that the highest death rates were found among the most sedentary individuals, without regard to weight. And this same study found that, among the physically fit, those who were "overweight" according to government health guidelines enjoyed significantly lower mortality rates than equally fit but "ideally thin" persons. (In this study, middle-aged physically fit women of average height weighing 146 pounds or more had almost half the mortality rate of equally fit women of the same height who weighed 115 pounds or less.) Similarly, a 1999 Cooper Institute study involving twenty-two thousand men found the highest death rate among sedentary men with waist measurements under thirty-four inches, while the lowest death rate was found among fit men with waist measurements of forty inches or more. A 1995 Blair study found that improved fitness (i.e., going from "unfit" to "fit"), with the latter requiring a level of exercise equivalent to going for a brisk half-hour walk four or five times per week, reduced subsequent mortality rates by 50%. The reduced mortality rates associated with improved fitness were not dependent on weight loss: Indeed, a decrease in BMI was associated with a slightly increased mortality risk. Glenn Gaesser points out that "Blair's findings indicate increasing fitness is far more important than decreasing BMI in terms of reducing mortality rates. It is also worth noting," Gaesser adds, "that Blair's data shows that the reduction in mortality rates associated with increasing aerobic fitness is linearly related to BMI: In other words, large people benefit the most from each increment of improved fitness. This is all the more reason to advocate fitness and physical activity as primary goals, not weight loss." As Blair himself puts it, Americans have "a misdirected obsession with weight and weight loss. The focus is all wrong. It's fitness that is the key."

Blair's work regarding the importance of fitness and activity levels confirms and extends that of other researchers. Ralph Paffenbarger's Harvard Alumni Study has found the lowest mortality rates among men who have *gained* the most weight since college, while also expending at least 2,000 calories per week in vigorous physical activities. The Behavioral Risk Factor Surveillance System, a large-scale study from the early 1990s, found that a lack of physical activity was a much better predictor of cardiovascular disease mortality than BMI. And a 2002 study of nearly ten thousand Puerto Rican men found that even modest amounts of physical activity had large health benefits for men across all weight ranges. This study found no correlation of any kind between "overweight" (BMI 25 to 29.9) and early mortality when physical activity was taken into account; furthermore, the authors found that "the likelihood of premature death among men who were obese (BMI 30+) did not reach statistical significance, especially after adjusting for other risk factors [such as sedentary lifestyle]." Thinness, on the other hand (BMI less than 18.5), had a strong correlation with early mortality, even after excluding men with preexisting coronary disease and everyone who died within three years of entry into the study.

The Puerto Rican study helps confirm a key element of Blair's work: that even modest amounts of physical activity are extremely beneficial to health, for people in all weight ranges. Blair has found that, to move into the category that offers most of the benefits associated with metabolic fitness, people need merely to engage in some moderately strenuous combination of daily physical activities equivalent to going for a brisk half-hour walk. In sum, the work done by Blair and others indicates that when obesity researchers have described the supposed health risks of fat, what they have really been doing is using fat as a proxy—and a poor one at that—for factors that actually do have a profound effect on health and mortality: aerobic fitness and physical activity.

Indeed, whether people are active or sedentary has very little to do with their weight. "In studies that divide up their subject pools according to physical activity levels," Gaesser told me, "the difference in average BMI between the most sedentary and the most active subject groups is never more than one or two BMI units, and usually less. This means that regular physical activity may be 'worth' only five to ten pounds of lower weight, at most." Gaesser also points out that while intervention studies designed to get sedentary people to become active almost always produce significant improvements in health, they almost never produce significant weight loss. The results of a recent study that involved getting "overweight" women to expend 2,000 calories per week through structured exercise are typical: After sixteen months of daily endurance activities, the study produced a total average weight loss of 1 pound among these women. Such results suggest that trying to get people to become active *for the purpose of making them thin* makes little sense.

The prosecution in the case against fat, by focusing obsessively

on a characteristic that, except in the most extreme instances, appears
to have little or no independent health significance, and that indeed
is something that most people cannot in the long run do anything
about, is obscuring the fact that the bulk of the medical evidence indicates that the health benefits of being physically active are almost
wholly independent of whether becoming active leads to any weight
loss. Yet the case against fat is based on the assumption that the
main point of becoming more physically active is to lose weight, even
though most people who become more active will not in the long run
become significantly thinner. This assumption ends up conveying a
false and destructive message to a nation in which somewhere around
three-quarters of the adult population engages in no significant physical activity of any kind.

Dieting, diet drugs, and sedentary lifestyle are just three of the
many variables that may well end up accounting for most or all of
whatever ill health can be found among some groups of heavier-than-
average persons. Consider, for example, the profound effects wealth
and poverty have on health, and then consider that, despite the striking correlation in contemporary America between increasing weight
and decreasing social class, almost none of the studies that purport to
measure the health risks of fat even attempt to control for this factor.
In short, as Glenn Gaesser points out, "as of 2002 there has not been
a single study that has truly evaluated the effects of weight alone on
health, which means that 'thinner is healthier' is not a fact, but an un-
substantiated hypothesis for which there is a wealth of evidence that
suggests the reverse."

Never Mind the Evidence:
Proceed with the Execution

As we have seen, the case against fat is based on four premises: that
everyone outside a very narrow weight range (a range that as of De-
cember 2002 did not include 80% of the American adult population)
is facing serious health risks; that the health problems seen outside
this narrow range are caused by being outside it; that those whose
weight falls above this range will eliminate their excess risk by getting
rid of their excess weight; and that there is some safe and effective
method available for achieving this goal. As we have also seen, these

premises are poorly supported, not supported at all, or flatly contra-
dicted by the available evidence. Most groups of people categorized as
"overweight" and "obese" do not suffer from poorer health or higher
mortality than "ideal weight" individuals. In many of the largest-scale
studies, groups of people currently categorized as overweight have better mortality statistics than anyone else. The bulk of the epidemiological evidence suggests that it is more dangerous to be 5 pounds
"underweight" than 75 pounds "overweight." The positive correlations
between disease and higher-than-average weight are quite problematic, and in any case are offset by similar correlations between equally
serious diseases and lower-than-average weight. There is essentially no
evidence that significant long-term weight loss improves health, and
quite a bit of evidence that short-term weight loss followed by weight
regain harms it. After more than a century of efforts to find a "cure" for
obesity, the medical profession has yet to find a safe method of permanent weight loss that is effective for more than a very small minority of
the seventy million Americans who are trying to lose weight on any
given day. And the tenuous connection between weight and health
tends to disappear altogether when factors other than weight are taken
into account.

In other words, upon closer inspection, every aspect of the case
against fat simply falls apart. Yet the collapse of this case raises all
sorts of further questions. None of the evidence I have laid out in this
chapter is particularly new; or rather, the many new pieces of evidence
I have cited simply confirm and amplify what the medical literature
has been suggesting for decades. Indeed, every assertion I have made
for the defense in the case against fat reflects the opinions of a host of
doctors, scientists, eating disorder specialists, psychologists, historians, sociologists, and other critics who for many years now have been
pointing out that the war against fat is both scientifically baseless and
socially destructive. From obesity researchers such as Glenn Gaesser,
Paul Ernsberger, Ancel Keys, Reubin Andres, Hilda Bruch, Wayne
Callaway, Steven Blair, Elizabeth Barrett-Conner, Janet Polivy, Paul
Askew, and Susan Wooley, to eating disorder specialists such as David
Garner and Joanne Ikeda, to historians of America's weight obsession
such as Hillel Schwartz and Roberta Seid, to social critics of that obsession such as Richard Klein and Laura Fraser, to feminist critics of
our absurdly restrictive body ideals such as Naomi Wolf, Kim Chernin,
Susan Bordo, and Susie Orbach, there has been no shortage of erudite

and eloquent voices crying out that the case against fat is based on an invidious combination of junk science and cultural neuroses. Yet the question remains: Why does the evidence seem to make so little difference in the prosecution of this particular case?

In his book *The Culture of Fear: Why Americans Are Afraid of the Wrong Things*, sociologist Barry Glassner explores why particular fears and anxieties capture our collective imagination. As Glassner demonstrates, it isn't a simple matter of being afraid of big risks and indifferent toward small ones. Building on the work of the eminent anthropologist Mary Douglas, Glassner argues that certain (often quite small) risks get selected for special emphasis "either because they offend the basic moral principles of society or because they enable criticism of disliked groups." Glassner also argues that another reason why Americans "harbor so many misbegotten fears is that immense power and money await those who tap into our moral insecurities and supply us with symbolic substitutes." As we shall see, these insights have great relevance to America's increasingly intense fear of fat.

Why are Americans so afraid of the generally small health risks associated with above-average weight, while remaining comparatively indifferent to the much larger health risks associated with being a man, or poor, or black, or for that matter unusually thin? To answer that question, we must look beyond the science of "obesity." We must approach the otherwise inexplicable social success of the case against fat, in the face of so much evidence, as a cultural and political phenomenon, as well as a fascinating chapter in the history of science. Understanding the bankruptcy of the scientific case against fat is an indispensable first step on that journey, but it is only the first step. The rest of this book is dedicated to exploring why, in America today, people of more than average weight are considered guilty until proven innocent—or rather are found guilty again and again, no matter what the evidence might say.

2

The World Turned Upside Down

FROM A STRICTLY ECONOMIC PERSPECTIVE, the market for the provision of medical care suffers from two almost unavoidable defects. First, effective treatments eliminate demand by curing the customers who purchase them. Second, ineffective treatments also tend to eliminate demand, either because, in the case of fatal diseases, customers who purchase such treatments die off, or because, in the case of nonfatal conditions, customers will normally choose not to treat the condition, once it becomes clear the treatment is ineffective.

From the perspective of a profit-maximizing medical and pharmaceutical industry, then, the ideal disease would be one that never killed those who suffered from it, that could not be treated effectively, and that doctors and their patients would nevertheless insist on treating anyway. Luckily for it, the American health-care industry has discovered (or rather invented) just such a disease. It is called "obesity."

The reasons why the disease of obesity doesn't kill those who suffer from it and why it remains impossible to cure are one and the same: Because it doesn't exist. "Obesity" is the name that medical science has given to that level of increasing body mass that, in and of itself, has significant negative consequences for a person's health. The problem with this definition is that, subject to exceptions at the extreme statistical margin, medical science has not been able to determine the existence of such a level, let alone fix its precise location.

Suppose it were discovered that people who owned at least six pairs of blue jeans also tended to be more sedentary than people who did not. Suppose further that this former group suffered from marginally poorer health than average. Now suppose that, for many years, the medical profession's response to these facts was to attempt to get sedentary people who owned lots of blue jeans to get rid of those pants. Finally, after several decades of almost complete failure, a new generation of researchers comes up with the idea of more or less forgetting about the blue jeans, and instead trying to get this group of people to be less sedentary. The results are startling: Basically, this new research demonstrates that you can own many pairs of blue jeans, and, as long as you are not sedentary, you will still be in far better health than people who are sedentary, even if such people own no blue jeans at all. Furthermore, you will be as healthy as active people who don't own any blue jeans.

Under such circumstances, one would think that the medical profession would be forced to admit that it had spent several decades operating on the basis of a fundamentally mistaken assumption. Owning blue jeans, after all, turns out to bear no causal relationship to poor health whatsoever. The correlation between the two was—like the vast majority of such correlations—almost wholly coincidental ("almost wholly" because it turns out that a tiny percentage of people own so many clothes that this fact in itself appears to cause such persons to be sedentary). The "disease" of Leviosity, or whatever it had been called, would now be recognized as a largely imaginary phenomenon.

Except for the business about the medical profession owning up to its mistakes, the above analogy describes the current state of obesity research. Now that confounding variables such as activity levels are at last being taken into account, researchers have discovered that, except for the most extreme cases, the apparent relationship between body mass and health—which was weak to begin with—is in most instances random.

However, there is still a fifty-billion-dollar-per-year industry dedicated to convincing Americans that if they don't get rid of their blue jeans they will be severely endangering their health. This industry isn't going to go away just because the flimsy scientific rationales it has constructed to justify its existence are now less plausible than ever before. Given that the most crucial public justification for the industry's existence continues to be the supposedly devastating health effects of blue jeans, it is safe to predict the industry will do everything in its power to fund medical research that keeps attempting to validate an increasingly implausible hypothesis.

This, too, is a good analogy for what has happened to the obesity debate in America. As Laura Fraser documents in her invaluable book *Losing It: False Hopes and Fat Profits in the Diet Industry*, many mainstream obesity researchers suffer from what she calls "thinking disorders." Basically, obesity research in America is funded by the diet and drug industry, that is, the economic actors who have the most to gain from the conclusion that being fat is a disease that requires aggressive treatment (less than 1% of the federal health research budget is dedicated to obesity issues). And such support goes far beyond the direct funding of studies. "Diet and pharmaceutical companies," Fraser emphasizes, "influence every step along the way of the scientific process. They pay for the ads that keep obesity journals publishing. They underwrite medical conferences, flying physicians around the country expense-free and paying them large lecture fees to attend."

Not only do obesity researchers depend on the diet industry to fund the bulk of their expenses: Many of these same researchers have direct financial relationships with the companies whose products they are evaluating. Indeed, Fraser describes several instances in which prominent researchers failed to acknowledge they had a financial stake in the research they were conducting and evaluating:

> Richard Wurtman, the MIT researcher whose company, Interneuron Pharmaceuticals, owns the patent to the obesity drug dexfenfluramine was frequently quoted in the media as an expert on the drug prior to its approval, foretelling its rosy possibilities, without any mention of his financial involvement. Louisiana State University obesity researcher George Bray presented his study on thigh cream without divulging that he'd already licensed the formula to the stuff to three companies.

Among other vignettes, Fraser details how a panel of obesity researchers published an article in *JAMA* purporting to provide a neutral evaluation of the benefits and risks of low-calorie liquid diets, while failing to reveal that several of the authors had direct financial ties to one of the largest manufacturers of such diets. Even those who are appropriately skeptical of the sometimes questionable relationship between academic research and the for-profit industries that help support it might find themselves taken aback by some of Fraser's revelations. For example, when she asked one researcher, who has condemned dieting as ineffectual and psychologically damaging, to comment on the policies of a well-known commercial weight loss program that pays him to sit on its scientific policy board, Fraser reports he replied (not for attribution), "What can I say? I'm a consultant for them."

The distorting effects of such factors help account for the otherwise inexplicable insistence of various obesity researchers that, despite the literally hundreds of articles in the medical literature questioning the existence of a causal relationship between increasing weight and ill health, there is in fact a consensus among scientists regarding the health risks of "excess" weight. For example, when I asked him to comment on Walter Willett's and Meir Stampfer's recent claim that "a strong international consensus among scientists" exists that a BMI of 25 and over is a major health risk, obesity researcher Paul Ernsberger pointed out that such claims are based on reports issued by groups like the World Health Organization and the NIH Obesity Task Force. "The WHO panel consisted entirely of physicians who run weight loss clinics," he told me. "Many of these clinics are largely dedicated to prescribing weight loss pills. The NIH Obesity Task Force, as I pointed out in a letter published in *JAMA*, consisted almost entirely of people running weight loss clinics." Ernsberger emphasizes that "this is a more fundamental conflict of interest than taking a few drug company checks. This is a conflict involving livelihood. The NIH and WHO assemble panels of doctors and psychologists who have dedicated their clinical practices to promoting weight loss. Indeed, in their reply to my letter in *JAMA*, the NIH has explained that their very definition of an obesity expert is "someone who runs a weight loss clinic." These people, Ernsberger notes, "are then asked to objectively evaluate the threat posed by obesity and the benefit provided by the clinics they run. In no other area of medicine are practitioners of a completely unrecognized specialty given such free rein to set their own ground rules."

Given these pervasive structural distortions, it is surprising that obesity research seems to have remained largely free of outright fraud. Despite research agendas framed to pursue a preordained conclusion— that obesity is a disease and that weight loss is an appropriate treatment for that disease—the data obesity researchers have actually compiled has made that conclusion increasingly difficult to defend. In the face of this fact, several prominent researchers, including Reubin Andres, Steven Blair, Elizabeth Barrett-Conner, Paul Ernsberger, Glenn Gaesser, Paul Haskew, Janet Polivy, Ancel Keys, Wayne Callaway, and Susan Wooley have ended up simply rejecting that conclusion outright. But a majority of the best-known obesity researchers continue to cling to the field's fundamental organizing principle (fat is a disease; weight loss is the cure) by employing two basic strategies: denial and distortion.

The first strategy manifests itself when researchers present their data in a straightforward manner, but then draw conclusions that clearly do not follow from their own description of their data. The typical piece of obesity research in America today can often be abstracted as follows: "We investigated the effects of diet treatment X on obese subjects. The effects included numerous adverse side effects. On average, the subjects gained all the weight they lost back, plus more, and their overall health was worse after undergoing treatment X than it was prior to the treatment. On the basis of this data, we conclude that obese persons ought to undergo treatment X (or perhaps an improved version of it)."

This is a parody, but not a very gross one. The last sentence in this hypothetical abstract illustrates what dissident obesity researcher Susan Wooley has called "the P.S. phenomenon." These are conclusions at the end of an article that ignore the evidence just presented by the article itself that dieting does more harm than good. Despite their own article's evidence, the authors will conclude that "overweight" people (again, for a woman of average height this means 146 pounds) should diet anyway. Such conclusions, Wooley says, can be interpreted as a coded message to the diet and drug industry: "P.S. Fund me again."

Numerous studies published in prestigious medical journals have come to similarly irrational conclusions. My favorite is a recent study that concludes the majority of weight variance is unalterably genetic, that this fact means most dieters will be "cyclic" (yo-yo) weight losers and gainers, and that weight cycling increases mortality. And the lesson the authors draw from their own data? "Most of the obesity research community has deemed such data [on the risks of weight loss] compelling—but not enough to state that weight-loss attempts by obese people are dangerous . . . Nowadays it is not uncommon to hear 'Diets don't work.' In fact, diets do work. It is prescriptions to diet that fail, because patients usually do not follow them." A better illustration of rampaging cognitive dissonance, as well as of the classic "the operation was a success but the patient died" line of argument, would be difficult to find.

As we have seen, such conclusions can be explained by the economic structure of obesity research. As a practical matter, obesity research must be funded either by the weight loss industry or by government grants. Government grant money is supposed to ameliorate the obviously distorting effects that arise when a big pharmaceutical firm is paying researchers to do work that will justify the tens or hundreds of millions of dollars the firm has invested in developing a particular "cure" for the "disease" of a higher-than-average weight. Yet grant money is scarce, and the process for securing it extremely competitive. One prominent obesity researcher described to me why so many people in the field seriously exaggerate the known health risks associated with weight. "The threat to careers may be most important of all. It's more than just being proved wrong," this researcher told me. "When you apply for a grant (to the NIH, for example) you have to make a strong case for funding by explaining the significance of the research." The researcher then asked me which of the following scenarios in the "significance" section of a grant I thought was most likely to produce a successful application:

1. "Though it is difficult to establish the independent contribution of obesity to morbidity and mortality, and it appears that lifestyle factors—such as poor diet and lack of physical activity—pose far greater health risks, we nevertheless request funding to study obesity as a matter of scientific curiosity, and also to assess whether it might be more prudent to get fat people fit rather than to get them thin."

Or:

2. "Obesity kills at least three hundred thousand Americans every year, and mathematical models of the obesity epidemic predict that within fifty years every man, woman and child in America will be overweight or obese."

"It's in the best interest of many people to portray obesity in the worst way possible," this researcher told me. "They get their funding, and it goes on and on. Since many of these researchers are connected to the highest-profile journals (such as *JAMA* and the *New England Journal of Medicine*), they are the ones who get the most media attention."

Indeed, some of the highest-profile obesity research appears beset by more insidious problems than merely exaggerating the health risks associated with increasing weight in order to secure funding. Certain prominent researchers cannot seem to resist the temptation to manipulate their data in ways that go beyond dubious interpretations of otherwise accurate statistics. Another well-known obesity researcher sketches a disturbing picture of how studies sometimes end up producing conclusions that at least superficially support the alarmist messages that benefit the interests of the authors of the studies, and of the weight loss industry in general. "What you see in a lot of these studies," this researcher told me, "is extensive manipulation of the subject base, a.k.a., 'data trimming.'"

I was first clued into this subject in the context of the famous Framingham study. Two reports on the impact of weight from the Framingham study appeared in *JAMA*. One showed no impact from overweight and only a slight effect from obesity, but a strong risk associated with underweight. I have a copy of some of the raw data tables from the government printing office, and they support this interpretation. The second paper appeared a couple of years later. It showed mortality risk increasing linearly with BMI. Why the differing conclusion? The answer, I believe, lies in a subtle statistic: the number of subjects. The data showing no harmful effect from overweight used all five thousand subjects. The later report used less than half the total number of subjects, and was very fuzzy regarding why it excluded the majority of the data pool. It's almost as if the authors excluded most of the "fat and healthy" and "sick and thin" subjects, leaving only the "fat and sick" and the "thin and healthy."

This researcher then went on to critique the methods of two of the most prominent people in the field.

[These two researchers] always exclude a large proportion of their study subjects. When they give a reason, it's usually that the subjects have a particular disease, or they have lost weight in the past ten years. (Another favorite is to exclude current smokers, conveniently overlooking the fact that ex-smokers are still at increased risk, and are almost invariably fatter than never-smokers.) But excluding certain subjects from consideration undermines the ability to *generalize* the results (anybody remember Statistics 101?). If you exclude everyone who has a disease, then your conclusions apply only to healthy people, and not to anyone who is ill. If you exclude everyone who has lost weight recently, then your conclusions apply only to weight-stable people. This means that [these two researchers'] weight guidelines, if they apply to anyone, only apply to people who are in perfect health and have a stable weight. The problem is that the guidelines are mainly applied to people who are not healthy, because these are the people coming into the doctor's office and getting the "lose weight or die" lecture.

The researcher then went on to give a detailed description of a recent study involving these authors, in which more than 20 percent of the subject pool ended up being excluded for various reasons. The study did not reveal any data regarding the excluded subjects, other than the criteria for exclusion, which, according to this researcher, "included some fairly benign conditions," with no explanation given for the exclusion criteria. "The problem I have with this is that the list of diseases used as grounds for exclusion ends up being unique for every paper [these authors publish]," this researcher said. "The amount of weight loss needed for exclusion, and the number of years in the study prior to death as a ground for exclusion also vary from report to report," the researcher added.

Why does this trouble me? What do I imagine is behind this "custom tailoring" of the data analysis? Well, imagine that your boss has demanded that you return a particular result from the data. You would run many different analyses. "Let's try excluding people with disease X. Is obesity harmful yet? No? Let's try excluding people with disease Y. Does omitting people who have lost 50 pounds give us our answer? No? Let's try 25 pounds, or

10." By running hundreds of different possible combinations of exclusion criteria, it is possible to edit your subject base in such a way as to support almost any result. Whatever happened to reporting the results from the group you originally enlisted in the study? In clinical trials, this sort of data trimming would get you in real trouble! Why is it tolerated only for studies of obesity? At the very least, these authors should be required to provide the results from their excluded subjects.

Unfortunately, it appears that as the case for the proposition that fat kills becomes weaker, these sorts of distortions have, if anything, become more common. Obesity researchers, after all, are only human; and there is no reason to believe their instinct for self-preservation (in this instance professional self-preservation) is any weaker than anybody else's. Indeed, a dispassionate analysis of the medical literature leads to the conclusion that, in a culture that considered fat to be as desirable as we consider slenderness to be, it is likely that being *thin* would be considered a massive health risk, while the health risks associated with increasing weight would be minimized or ignored. More to the point, within such a world turned upside down, the case for the health risks of what would be characterized as the "disease" of "emaciation" could in fact be made with less distortion of the data than has been employed by those who exaggerate the health risks of "obesity" in America today.

Consider what such a world would look like. First of all, we need to imagine a culture in which fat is associated with sexual desirability, wealth, and status, and thinness is considered both aesthetically disgusting and a sign of poverty and lack of self-respect. Strictly speaking, it isn't necessary to *imagine* such a culture: This is in fact a fairly accurate description of the United States during the last few decades of the nineteenth century, and indeed of many other cultures, both past and present. In West Africa today, beauty pageants feature contestants who would be considered markedly "obese" in the United States; many of the young women who represent the pinnacle of female beauty in these cultures weigh more than 200 pounds. In this regard, contemporary West Africa is quite similar to the United States in the 1890s, when the 200-pound actress Lillian Russell was considered the undisputed beauty of her time. Historically speaking, far more cultures have mirrored contemporary West Africa and America in the latter half of the nineteenth century, than have resembled the United States today, where an almost unprecedented ideal of thinness reigns supreme.

If the American elites had maintained the same attitude toward fat throughout the twentieth century that they displayed during the Gilded Age, we can be sure the contemporary science of body mass studies would look radically different. For one thing, the term "obesity" would either not exist or would be reserved for those extremes of body fat (those that cause almost complete immobility) at which an adverse effect on health becomes undeniable. Medical research projects looking into the relationship between body mass and health would have assumed from the very beginning that being too thin was a significant health risk—and sure enough, that is precisely what their studies would reveal (indeed, in the majority of large-scale epidemiological surveys, the thinnest cohorts have the shortest life expectancy).

Medical researchers specializing in the study of the detrimental effects of "emaciation" would soon compile a long list of diseases, including lung, stomach, and breast cancer; anemia; osteoporosis; hip fracture; and almost all the major respiratory ailments, whose prevalence correlated with (and was therefore assumed to be caused by) a lack of adequate supplies of body fat. Every month, the various journals dedicated to emaciation studies would publish yet more articles illustrating the undeniable correlation between thinness and a host of crippling and even fatal conditions.

At the intersection of science and economics, insurance companies would have noticed early on that their thinnest policyholders tended to die sooner than any others, and would have produced height and weight charts emphasizing this fact. The government, reacting to a medical and economic consensus that thinness kills, would promulgate body mass recommendations that would characterize a BMI in the middle to upper 20s as "ideal" (this, again, actually correlates with the findings of several of the largest epidemiological surveys), and would recommend that all people with BMI figures below 20, as well as those with thinness-correlated health problems and BMI figures below 25, take aggressive steps to try to gain weight.

Under such cultural conditions, of course, the vast majority of prominent public figures would be fat. Thin politicians would realize they had no realistic chance of gaining the highest offices if they could not gain and keep on a significant amount of weight. Thin actors, and especially thin actresses, would be condemned to playing a few stereotypical roles—roles that would almost always focus on the comedic or pathetic nature of thinness. The average fashion model would weigh 200 pounds. Thin job candidates would almost always lose out to similarly qualified fat competitors; and thin single people would despair of finding mates who didn't look like Kate Moss or Keanu Reeves—two people who would remain completely anonymous in the context of this parallel world.

We can also be certain that, in such an America, an industry would arise, and grow to multibillion-dollar proportions, dedicated to helping thin people gain weight. Despite massive investments in food products and drugs designed to help people suffering from "emaciation" put on pounds, most such efforts would fail (data on the force-feeding of prisoners indicates that it is nearly as difficult for thin people to keep weight on as it is for fat people to take it off). Thin people would be encouraged to blame themselves for failing to develop bodies more in keeping with the cultural ideal, and as a consequence they would suffer from depression, which in turn would cause them to become even thinner than they would have been if they had never tried to gain weight in the first place.

This in turn would lead to ever-more histrionic warnings from the government, the medical establishment, and the pharmaceutical industry (the latter would be focusing much of its research on finding a magic weight-gain pill) that America was "starving to death." Eating disorders such as anorexia nervosa and bulimia would, of course, be extraordinarily rare; but such instances of these conditions as did arise would draw enormous publicity, and would be highlighted as prime examples of the "emaciation epidemic" sweeping through America. Meanwhile, millions of Americans, especially adolescent girls and young women, would on a daily basis ingest the highest-fat foods available, and avoid all exercise, in a desperate attempt to gain control over their stubbornly thin bodies. A succession of Surgeon Generals would declare the emaciation epidemic the nation's number one public health crisis. The rich would get fatter; the poor would get thinner; and public officials and public opinion makers would wring their (invariably plump) hands in despair.

Eventually, a group of unorthodox emaciation researchers would begin to question the standard view of emaciation. They would emphasize that, while extreme levels of emaciation were no doubt unhealthy, there was little evidence to suggest that people with BMI figures of

18.5 to 24.9 had any worse health than those in the supposedly "ideal" range of 25 to 29.9. Furthermore, they would point out that the health problems associated with high levels of fat—which even the orthodox emaciation researchers admitted existed at extremely high levels of body mass—often began to be fairly marked for people with fashionably fat BMI figures, not merely at the greatest extremes of fat. These researchers would also turn a skeptical eye on the weight-gaining industry, pointing to the plentiful data that indicated attempts to gain weight did more harm than good, and that many of the health problems suffered by thin people could be traced directly to their unsuccessful efforts to become fatter.

Yet the real revolution in emaciation studies would not begin until emaciation researchers started to include confounding variables in their previously simplistic data sets, such as smoking and exercise. Once these factors were taken into account, it would begin to become clear that, contrary to the conventional wisdom, there was actually very little relationship between thinness and poor health, except at the most extreme levels. "Fitness, not fatness" would become the motto of the new breed of emaciation researchers, and of their growing number of allies among psychologists, gaining disorder specialists, and thin activists, all of whom would have had years of experience dealing with the consequences of the fear and loathing inspired in America by the very thought of a thin body.

Given the degree of fear and loathing inspired by the very thought of a fat body in America today, it is important to emphasize that all of the medical information in the counterfactual world I have just sketched is itself quite factual. The point is, if such facts were viewed through a cultural prism that celebrated fat and condemned thinness, it would soon become all too "obvious" that thinness killed, and that maintaining an appropriately high percentage of body fat was largely a matter of willpower and lifestyle. Doctors, bureaucrats, and journalists would be happy to inform dissenters at every turn that everyone knew thinness was a pathological condition, if not an outright symptom of moral turpitude. "Nowadays it is not uncommon to hear 'gaining weight doesn't work,'" articles seeking a cure for emaciation would proclaim. But this, we would be assured, was simply not the case. "In fact, gaining weight does work. It is prescriptions to gain weight that fail, because patients do not follow them."

On the other hand, given our culture's hunger for simple answers to complex questions, it's also important to emphasize that I am not saying that there actually *is* an emaciation epidemic in America. It is true that, when one considers the extent of the damage done by the eating disorders from which at least eight million Americans currently suffer, as well as the often devastating health consequences of yo-yo dieting, it would be more accurate to say that, in contemporary America, there is little question that attempting to lose weight causes many more health problems than fat does. Indeed, it's remarkable that larger people in America do not, on the whole, have significantly worse health than thin people, given the stresses to which the culture subjects their psyches and their bodies.

But ultimately such generalizations about the health consequences of weight do more harm than good. Medicine has only recently become anything like a science; and, in the realm of public health policy, medical knowledge and especially its limitations are so often distorted by political and cultural factors that the scientific elements of the discipline can be easily buried under the weight of ideology, cultural fashion, and outright prejudice. The absurd notion that something as complex as an individual human being's health can be adequately gauged, or even generalized about, by determining where he or she fits on something as crude as a body mass index scale is a remnant of a level of medical knowledge (or rather ignorance) that had very little to do with science in any useful sense of that much-abused word.

"Emaciation," then, is just as imaginary a disease as "obesity." Neither exists in the same sense that lung cancer or diabetes exists. Both are (or, in the case of the former, would be) conceptual artifacts of a culture whose need to control the world and the people in it is so intense that it has been driven to such preposterous conclusions as the idea that millions of unique individuals should all weigh within 10 pounds of an imaginary ideal weight. In fact, as we have seen, there is no valid medical reason why two women of the same height cannot weigh 100 and 200 pounds respectively, while both maintain optimum cardiovascular and metabolic fitness, and excellent overall health.

There is no medical reason why this should not be the case: But, as we are about to see, there are enormously powerful cultural, political, and economic forces that ensure we do our best to make sure one of these women will remain miserable about her "disease." This disease, she is reminded constantly, is as disgusting as leprosy. Furthermore, it is a disease that she is told she could rid herself of at any time, if only she had the willpower (and the money) to subject herself to the latest in the long line of cures proffered by the medical and pharmacological establishment.

It takes only a little imagination to envision a world turned upside down, in which this persecuted woman weighs 100 pounds, rather than 200. Such an exercise is worth undertaking, if only to remind us of the strange contingencies that determine such things as the cultural definition of an ideal body. Indeed, one might say that there but for the grace of the culture that gives us *Vogue* magazine (and the science of obesity studies) go Calista Flockhart and Kate Moss.

PART II

FAT CULTURE

He had still, he reflected, not learned the ultimate secret. He understood how; *he did not understand* why.

—GEORGE ORWELL, *1984*

3

Fear and Loathing in Los Angeles

THE COVER of the March 2000 issue of *Harper's* magazine features a photograph of an artwork entitled *Sundae 1*, by Jeanne Dunning. The photograph is of the head and shoulders of a person of indeterminate gender, lying on his or her back. The person's face is completely smothered by an artfully stacked mound of whipped cream, topped with a cherry.

The cover story the photograph is meant to entice readers to sample is "Let Them Eat Fat: The Heavy Truths About American Obesity," by Greg Critser. This essay is in many ways representative of the sort of reportage regarding weight-related issues now appearing on a daily basis in the nation's major newspapers and large-circulation magazines. The basic thesis of such stories is almost always the same: Americans are eating themselves to death. Yet readers of these stories who remain willing to look just below their surface of alarmist claims and distorted statistics will often find evidence of things a good deal more disturbing than the number of calories in a Double Whopper with cheese. In this regard, "Let Them Eat Fat" is an especially revealing document. Indeed, its author's unusual candor makes this essay an excellent introduction to the underlying cultural sources of our increasingly intense obsession with the dietary habits and waistlines of our fellow citizens.

The essay itself opens with what its author clearly intends to be a shocking and horrifying tableau: In the intensive care unit of the

University of Southern California's medical center in downtown Los Angeles, a twenty-two-year-old man whom Critser names "Carl" is being intubated, while surgeons "labor to save his life." Critser informs us that Carl weighs 500 pounds. The author then quotes the patient's mother: " 'Second time in three months,' [she] blurted out to me as she stood apart watching in horror. 'He had two stomach staplings, and they both came apart. Oh my God, my boy . . .' Her boy was suffocating in his own fat."

"Here . . . writhed a real-life epidemiological specter," notes the shocked and horrified author, employing a metaphor that suggests *Harper's* editors were not at the top of their games when this piece came across their desks. (As we shall see, neither were the magazine's fact checkers.)

The magazine's readers are never told what medical condition has occasioned this emergency. Given the assertions made in the rest of his essay, I suspect it may come as a surprise to the author to learn that "suffocating in your own fat" does not constitute a recognized medical diagnosis. More to the point, using "Carl's" unspecified medical problems to introduce a discussion of weight and public health is typical of the sorts of anxiety-provoking distortions employed by America's anti-fat warriors. Only a tiny percentage of the 135 million adult Americans who the government claims are "overweight" are anywhere near Carl's size. By focusing on the most extreme cases, those prosecuting the war on fat copy the drug war's most deceptive tactics: Just as the average American who our government labels a "drug abuser" is someone who smokes marijuana occasionally, the average American being harassed by our public health authorities about her supposedly unhealthy weight is a 150-pound woman, not a 500-pound man.

But leave all this aside for the moment. Critser goes on to cite the usual scare statistics about an "obesity epidemic" in America, before offering up a particularly choice quote from David Satcher. Satcher, who succeeded C. Everret Koop as Surgeon General, is perhaps even more unhinged on the subject of obesity than his fat-obsessed predecessor. "Today," Satcher solemnly intones to a gathering of federal bureaucrats and policymakers, "we see a nation of young people at serious risk of starting out obese and dooming themselves to the tough task of overcoming a serious illness."

The rhetorical stakes are then ratcheted even higher with a quote from William Dietz, the director of nutrition at the Centers for Disease Control (Critser employs the neat journalistic trick of always characterizing the most histrionic of his sources as "the most careful" and "normally reticent" experts): "This is an epidemic in the U.S. the likes of which we have not had before in chronic disease," Dietz says. Critser expands on this ridiculous claim—which any journalist armed with a scintilla of skepticism would recognize as exactly the sort of thing a CDC honcho angling for a bigger slice of the federal health research pie might say—with an even more preposterous observation of his own. "The cost [of obesity] to the general public health budget by 2020," Critser predicts, "will run into the hundreds of billions, making HIV look, economically, like a bad case of the flu." (An outbreak of influenza in 1918 killed between twenty and forty million people worldwide, including 675,000 Americans, but never mind.)

The essay goes on to frame its subject in a manner that—no doubt unintentionally—recalls Jonathan Swift's eighteenth-century masterpiece of satirical invective, "A Modest Proposal," in which Swift suggested that the Anglo-Irish ruling class should encourage the Irish poor to fatten up their children, and then sell them for slaughter: "How is it that we Americans, perhaps the most health-conscious of any people in the history of the world, and certainly the richest, have come to preside over the deadly fattening of our youth?" Critser asks.

Before getting to his answer, I should note that to this point "Let Them Eat Fat" has been fairly standard stuff. I simply never would have believed, before I began to study the issue of fat in America, how inaccurate most of the mainstream journalism regarding this issue actually is. Typical newspaper and magazine articles on fat are generally worse than worthless: Such stories tend to be nothing more than lemming-like compendia of various gross distortions, fed to a compliant media by those in the medical and pharmaceutical establishment who profit directly from the constant escalation of America's weight anxiety. (If stories on the drug war consisted mainly of rewrites of press releases from the White House's Office of Drug Policy, they would be about as reliable as the average journalistic foray into the war on fat.)

Readers of this *Harper's* article, and of the hundreds of pieces of journalism churned out annually that repeat its central claims, will never guess that there is a raging debate in the medical literature about whether "obesity" is even a useful concept. They will never be given a hint of the fact that, in the words of the editors of the *New*

England Journal of Medicine, the case for the claim that fat is a significant health risk is "limited, fragmentary and often ambiguous." They
are not going to be informed that far more Americans do serious damage to their health by attempting to lose weight than by gaining it. And
they will never hear of the powerful evidence gathered over the past
two decades that a lack of cardiovascular and metabolic fitness, not an
excess of fat, is the key to understanding ill health among *both* fat and
thin Americans.

No, most readers will come away from such articles with the belief
(as I did, when my knowledge of the subject came from similar sources)
that "obesity" is a major health risk in America, if not an outright epidemic disease—one that dwarfs AIDS in its potential to devastate the
children of the poor and the pocketbooks of the rich (more on that
particular connection in a moment).

Of course all of this is either greatly exaggerated or flatly untrue. I
ask readers to forgive a bit of repetition, intended to fight the reflexive
incredulity that, as a consequence of so much weight loss industry
propaganda, the following facts tend to elicit among even the best-
informed audiences: Weight is on the whole a poor predictor of health.
Even quite fat people have better health, on average, than fashionably
thin women. Fat active people have half the mortality rate of thin
sedentary people. Levels of physical activity are far better predictors of
health than body mass. Dieting does far more damage to health than
being fat. And so on.

You would never guess any of this from reading or viewing the vast
majority of stories published or broadcast about weight in the nation's
major media. Attempting to explain the causes of this remarkable level
of distortion is one of the aims of this book. One source of that distortion is the understandable hunger to find simple explanations for complex problems. Americans are on the whole pragmatic people who like
to believe problems have solutions, especially if these problems are
subjected to the rigors of "scientific policymaking." Simply assuming
that heavier people are less healthy than thin ones, and that the former would be healthier if they were thinner, makes it much easier
to draft nice, straightforward grant proposals, and to formulate nice,
unambiguous public health policies. (It's also a great way to secure
funding from pharmaceutical companies.) A close cousin of this phenomenon is the professional deformation that takes place when an en-

tire discipline is organized initially around a fundamentally mistaken assumption: in this case, the assumption at the core of obesity studies that higher than average weight is a significant independent health risk.

Another explanation, one illustrated well by the substance of the mainstream journalism discussing weight, is that almost all of us rely on the conventional wisdom regarding a particular subject for essentially all of our information about that subject. Unless we have some fairly specialized knowledge about X, our opinions about X will almost always reflect the opinions about X held by people like us. At bottom, journalists tend to believe what they believe about fat because what they believe about fat simply reflects the views about fat held by the people they know best—many of whom, of course, are other journalists. And even those among their circle who are not journalists will still tend to be people very much like them—upper-class, mostly white professionals who can for the most part be counted on to share the same basic beliefs as their journalist friends, spouses, and so on.

Given all this, it's hardly surprising that journalists will often come to an issue such as the relationship between weight and health with the point of view that will frame the researching and writing of their stories already firmly in place. Since most of their research will, by necessity, consist of reading the work of other journalists on this same issue, supplemented, perhaps, by new quotations from the very same experts and government agencies that were quoted in these previous stories, the new stories inevitably end up looking very much like the old ones.

I have no affection for conspiracy theories; and most popular accounts of how information gets interpreted and distorted by the media tend to be both too rationalistic and too conspiratorial. But I will say this: The experience of reading hundreds of articles about fat published in our nation's major media over the course of the last few years, while at the same time actually studying the primary scientific research regarding the subject, is something that can make theories of manufactured consent and the like begin to look fairly plausible. As the joke goes, a paranoid person is somebody who suspects what's really going on. Except that it isn't always a joke: Spend three years reading the scientifically spurious propaganda of the diet industry dressed up as "investigative journalism," and then get back to me.

Anyway, back to "Let Them Eat Fat." The most valuable feature of this essay is the relatively clear glimpse it provides into many of the emotions, ideological inclinations, and outright prejudices that help explain why we are beset by so many irresponsible public policies directed toward the issue of weight in America. This is, in a sense, to its author's credit. For Critser does not, like so many other writers on this subject, wholly repress any explicit acknowledgment of the more disturbing impulses that fuel the war on fat.

Critser thinks he has found, on the streets of Los Angeles, the answer to his question regarding how Americans can be so health-conscious and so fat at the same time. A recent article in *Glamour* magazine, written by a *Glamour* editor whose assignment was to go an entire week without weighing herself or counting calories (this was clearly meant to be perceived by the magazine's readership as a Herculean task) describes Los Angeles as a city where it's "illegal to sign a lease if you have a body fat percentage of more than 6%." That's one side of the city to be sure (the west side, more or less). But in what Critser describes as "the heart of the San Fernando Valley's burgeoning Latino population," the situation is quite different. It is here that Critser attends the opening of a new Krispy Kreme doughnut store, and witnesses scenes that he describes in something akin to the tone of a Victorian missionary confronting the savage rituals of the natives, somewhere deep within the heart of darkness.

Critser interviews the manager of the store, who touches on the elaborate marketing strategies that go into choosing the location of a new Krispy Kreme outlet: " 'The idea is simple—accessible but not convenient . . . We want them intent to get at least a dozen before they even think of coming in.' " Critser asks the manager who these prospective marketing targets might be. "He gestured to the stout Mayan doñas queuing around the building. 'We're looking for all the bigger families.' " "Bigger in size?" Critser asks with what appears to be an almost pornographic air of fascination. " 'Yeah.' [The manager's] eyes rolled, like little glazed crullers. *'Bigger in size.'* "

At this point I should say something about my own background. My parents came to the United States from Mexico in the year of my birth; my mother remained a Mexican citizen for twenty years after that; and I spoke only Spanish when I began going to school. All of which is to say that as a Mexican American, I'm naturally more attuned to the resonance of statements involving "stout Mayan doñas" than most of my fellow citizens. At the same time, however, I'm someone who has always been suspicious of identity politics in all of its forms, and who has said so repeatedly in print. Few things annoy me more than any sentence beginning "As a (Latino/gay/Asian/feminist etc.), I am offended by. . . ."

I mention all this to give some context to my reaction to what follows in Critser's essay—material whose full flavor cannot be appreciated without extensive quotation.

> At my local McDonald's, located in a lower-middle-income area of Pasadena, California, the supersize bacchanal goes into high gear at about 5 P.M., when the various urban caballeros, drywalleros, and jardineros get off from work and head for a quick bite. Mixed in is a sizeable element of young black kids traveling between school and home, their economic status apparent by the fact that they've walked instead of driven. Customers are cheerfully encouraged to "supersize your meal!" by signs saying, "If we don't recommend a supersize, the supersize is free!" For an extra seventy-nine cents, a kid ordering a cheeseburger, small fries and a small coke will get said cheeseburger plus a supersize Coke (42 fluid ounces versus 16, with free refills) and a supersize order of french fries (more than double the weight of a regular order). Suffice it to say that consumption of said meals is fast and, in almost every instance I observed, very complete.

Again, note the lurid tone: You would think the author had been watching teenagers exchange sexual favors for crack cocaine, given the text's mixture of salacious detail and horrified sanctimoniousness.

And that is not all. Critser goes on to agonize over the contents of the "jumbo dietetic horror" he has witnessed, and to describe the "endocrine warfare" he believes is sure to erupt in the bodies of the wretched refuse of our teeming shores who engage in such flagrant self-abuse. Then he really lets us know what he thinks:

> If childhood obesity truly is "an epidemic in the U.S. the likes of which we have not had before in chronic disease," then places like McDonald's and Winchell's Donut stores, with their

endless racks of glazed and creamy goodies, are the San Francisco bathhouses of said epidemic, the places where the high-
risk population indulges in high-risk behavior. Although open
around the clock, the Winchell's near my house doesn't get
rolling until seven in the morning, the Spanish-language talk
shows frothing in the background while an ambulance light whirls
atop the Coke dispenser. Inside, Mami placates Miguelito with
a giant apple fritter. Papi tells a joke and pours ounce upon
ounce of sugar and cream into his 20-ounce coffee. Viewed
through the lens of obesity, as I am inclined to do, the scene is
not so *feliz*.

By now, we might wonder, why hasn't the frantic author hurled
himself bodily between that giant apple fritter and poor little Miguelito,
or at least called the police? Indeed, at this point even the most anti-
PC Hispanic you can find might well want to ask the author a couple
of questions. Such as, did some urban caballero ride off with his girlfriend or something? And what is it with these skinny uptight Anglos,
anyway? Who exactly deputized them to be the fat police at their local
fast-food emporia?

Critser has an answer to these questions (or at least to the latter
one). His focus on the ethnicity of all these Mayan doñas and peripa-
tetic black kids and doughnut-crazed Mexicans has nothing whatsoever to do with the phenomenon of upper-class white people being
revolted by the sight of fat, working-class, non-white persons, possibly
of extra-national provenance, gorging themselves like animals in a vis-
cerally disgusting (but actually quite tasty—ever had a Krispy Kreme
doughnut?) bacchanal of forbidden treats. Oh no. He is merely sounding the alarm, in a desperate attempt to save these hopelessly simple
people from themselves.

"The obesity rate for Mexican-American children," the author informs us sternly, "is shocking." He returns to the scene of the ongoing
doughnut crime: "The lovely but very chubby little girl tending to
her schoolbooks . . . will begin puberty before the age of ten, launching her into a lifetime of endocrine bizarreness that will not only be
costly to treat but will be emotionally devastating as well." Critser
doesn't need to add that all this "bizarreness" will also give her a big
head start over all those anorexic (and therefore infertile) white girls in
the nicer parts of Pasadena, in the Darwinian struggle to produce the

next generations of (respectively) Krispy Kreme junkies and Diet Coke addicts.

To be fair, Critser doesn't really want to focus on what he calls "the inevitable divisiveness of race and gender." He wants to talk about the relationship between fat and social class. On this topic, he actually makes a good deal of sense. He notes that, in America today, the poor are fat and the rich are not—and he even considers the possibility that the rich would like to keep things that way. "In upscale corporate America," he notes, "being fat is taboo, a sure-fire career-killer. If you can't control your own contours, goes the logic, how can you control a budget and staff? Look at the glossy business and money magazines with their cooing profiles of the latest genius entrepreneurs: To the man, and the occasional woman, no one, I mean *no one*, is fat."

One would hope that a journalist confronting a situation such as this—in which a physical characteristic was being used to disenfranchise a significant portion of the citizenry from the upper echelons of money and power—would display a modicum of curiosity about whether the things the people with the money and power were saying about the supposed awfulness of that physical characteristic were actually true. But, at this moment in America, when it is no longer possible to observe that a glossy brochure contains no pictures of women, or nonwhites, without being expected to wonder if there's a legitimate reason for that absence, it is still possible—and indeed almost obligatory—to assume there is a good reason for excluding fat people.

It would be difficult to come up with a better illustration of the distorting power of the war on fat than Critser's explanation for why Americans—specifically poor and working-class Americans—are getting fatter, when being fat has so clearly become an enormous social disadvantage. According to Critser, it's because America's elites have been afraid to say or do anything to signal social disapproval of fat. Cowed by, among others, "a very vocal minority of super-obese female activists . . . the media, the academy, public health workers, and the government do almost nothing" to let Americans know that being fat is undesirable. This hypothesis, of course, is simply insane on its face.

In America today, it is impossible for anyone above the age of about five—recent news reports indicate that fat anxiety is becoming common among six- to eight-year-olds—to somehow miss the fact that power and privilege in all of its forms are associated with thinness, and, especially in the case of women, unhealthy extremes of thinness.

Go into any supermarket, look at any magazine rack, glance at any television screen, visit any movie theater, enter any office building, peruse any glossy entrepreneurial profile—indeed, walk down a city street with your eyes open, and you will get the message. What's amazing is that, as we have seen, Critser gets the message loud and clear when he recognizes that thinness and economic privilege are closely connected in our culture—and yet he instantly forgets this fact when he attempts to explain why the have-nots are getting fatter.

His thesis that "those with true cultural power, those in the academy and the publishing industry who have the ability to shape public opinion" have been so cowed by feminists and the like that they display a systematic "reluctance to face [the] facts" about fat is, under the circumstances, nothing less than bizarre. After all, Critser's essay itself manages to remain almost fact-free in regard to the obesity debate (indeed, he seems unaware there *is* a debate) precisely because it is a product of a cultural atmosphere in which investigative journalists writing for high-profile magazines have been so thoroughly brainwashed about the supposed health risks of fat that they don't bother to engage in the most cursory investigation of their topic.

Critser concludes on an apocalyptic note:

What do the fat, darker, exploited poor, with their unbridled primal appetites, have to offer us but a chance for we diet-and-shape-conscious folk to live vicariously? Call it boundary envy. Or, rather, boundary-free envy . . . Meanwhile, in the City of Fat Angels, we lounge through a slow-motion epidemic. Mami buys another apple fritter. Papi slams his second sugar and cream. Another young Carl supersizes and double supersizes, then supersizes again. Waistlines surge. Any minute now, the belt will run out of holes.

In his book *The Anatomy of Disgust*, William Ian Miller traces the ways in which that emotion is related to both fear and moral judgment. We become disgusted when what would otherwise remain mere contempt becomes enriched by, among other things, a fear of contamination: "We know when we are disgusted and we usually know when we are afraid. But the two are frequently co-experienced: thus the easiness and the justness of the collocation 'fear and loathing.' . . . Intense disgust invites fear to attend, because contamination is a frightful thing."

Indeed it is. As Miller points out, disgust "operates in a kind of miasmic gloom, in the realm of horror, in regions of dark unbelievability, and never too far away from the body's and, by extension, the self's interiors."

If one were forced to come up with a six-word explanation for the otherwise inexplicable ferocity of America's war on fat, it would be this: Americans think being fat is disgusting. It really is, on the most important cultural and political levels, as simple as that. Critser's article is merely an unusually clear example of the commonplace social process by which a visceral reaction is transmuted into an aesthetic judgment, which in turn becomes a series of (imaginary) facts about the relationship between weight and health.

Critser dismisses as "vulgar social psychology" the idea that hatred of fat might be driven by "our need for an identifiable outsider." Yet a few strokes of Occam's razor makes it evident that this is in fact a highly plausible explanation for the genesis of the sort of hysterical diatribe Critser himself produces, featuring as it does so much voyeuristic ogling of fat Mexicans enjoying giant apple fritters.

Fifty years ago, America was full of people that the social elites could look upon with something approaching open disgust: blacks in particular, of course, but also other ethnic minorities, the poor, women, Jews, homosexuals, and so on. (An example: I remember from my childhood in the 1970s that Polish jokes were a regular feature of Johnny Carson's *Tonight Show* monologue.) Yet over the last half-century, the classes of candidates available for open pariah status have gradually shrunk. This has become a problem on at least two levels. As many a vulgar social psychologist has (correctly) observed, societies need pariahs. In most cultures, some class of people is more or less required to play the role of those who make everybody else feel superior by comparison. Furthermore, the feelings of disgust elicited in others by traditional pariah-class individuals do not simply disappear as soon as it becomes unacceptable to express those feelings openly.

As *The Handbook of Obesity Studies* notes (Critser himself cites this precise quote): "In heterogeneous and affluent societies such as the United States, there is a strong inverse correlation of social class and obesity, particularly for females." In other words, on average, poor people in America are fat, and rich people are thin. A strong correlation also exists between obesity and ethnic minority status—one that goes beyond the class correlation itself. Particularly among African American women, changing class status does not appear to strongly influence obesity rates (in America, the demographic group with the highest obesity rate is that comprised of black women in their fifties). Critser notes this as well, and muses that some observers might claim "black women find affirmation for being heavy from black men, or believe themselves to be 'naturally' heavy." He then adds prissily that "such assertions do not change mortality statistics."

This last observation is really too much. As we have seen, Critser does not appear to have looked at (or at any rate understood) any mortality statistics whatsoever. If he had, he might have discovered that studies investigating the relationship between weight and health among African-American women have found no correlation between increasing weight and mortality among such women, even at very high levels of "obesity."

Yet ultimately all this is beside the point. The disgust the thin upper classes feel for the fat lower classes has nothing to do with mortality statistics, and everything to do with feelings of moral superiority engendered in thin people by the sight of fat people. Precisely because Americans are so repressed about class issues, the disgust the (relatively) poor engender in the (relatively) rich must be projected onto some other distinguishing characteristic. In 1853, an upper-class Englishman could be quite unself-conscious about the fact that the mere sight of the urban proletariat disgusted him. In 2003, any upper-class white American liberal would be horrified to imagine that the sight of say, a lower-class Mexican-American woman going into a Wal-Mart might somehow elicit feelings of disgust in his otherwise properly sensitized soul. But the sight of a fat woman—make that an "obese"— better yet a "morbidly [sic] obese" woman going into Wal-Mart . . . ah, that is something else again.

And, precisely because we live in a culture obsessed with fat hatred, the otherwise potentially disturbing fact that this woman, who often elicits feelings of disgust in white upper-class observers, also just happens to be poor and non-white can be dismissed by those observers as an irrelevant coincidence. (It's difficult to imagine a magazine such as Harper's publishing the sort of ethnic insults that fill

Critser's article in any context other than one in which those insults are aimed at fat people.)

At bottom, the reason upper-class Americans are so disgusted by, and terrified of, fat is that in this culture fat has the power to contaminate. Fat has the power, metaphorically speaking, to make us non-white and poor—and under current cultural conditions it is much easier for an upper-class white person to become fat than it is for him or her to become poor, let alone non-white.

Seen in this light, the almost pornographic quality of Critser's descriptions of fat people eating fast food begins to make sense. For what Critser calls "we diet-and-shape-conscious folk," a Krispy Kreme doughnut is not just a doughnut: It is a fetishistic, almost magical object, with the power to contaminate and transform those who allow themselves to be seduced by its quasi-erotic charms. Each bite of that doughnut, each moment of weakness that tempts us to supersize those fries, or to surrender to the orgiastic frenzy in which we imagine little Miguelito and the millions like him greedily ripping apart their enormous apple fritters, pushes us closer to death—and to something even worse.

In his studies of the comparative development of cultures, Jared Diamond has noted that as societies become more complex, they almost always become more sedentary, bureaucratic, and hierarchical. In America today, we are generally quite sensitive to the first two trends, while ignoring or denying the third. But who can deny that, in a nation where, as Critser himself puts it, "no one, and I mean *no one*" in the pages of the glossy magazines within which the elite project their image of themselves is anything like fat, the hierarchy of acceptable body types is becoming more rigid, exclusive, and well-defined than ever before?

The image on the cover of *Harper's* is not merely, in one sense, pornographic: It is fraught with implications of death. A colleague to whom I showed the image to illustrate the concept of "food porn" commented that it was also, as she put it, an image of "death by sundae." And indeed, when seen through the lens of the anxieties of the upper classes in America today—when seen through the eyes of we who are afraid of being enveloped, smothered, crushed, and, most of all, contaminated by the rippling mountains of fat cascading down the bodies of our social inferiors—the message of *Sundae I* becomes quite clear: Eat fat and die. Or worse yet: Become one of *them*.

4

Lost in the Supermarket

GUSTAVE FLAUBERT is supposed to have remarked that the only way to improve ice cream would be to make it a sin. As usual, American ingenuity has been up to the task.

I have before me an advertisement for "the Marble Slab Creamery Experience." Below these words is a photograph of a winsome lass, standing in front of a counter laden with bananas and pineapples. A come-hither smile on her face, she is thrusting an enormous ice cream cone straight out toward her audience. Virginal vanilla ice cream is piled up high about the ridges of a massive waffle cone. The ice cream itself is decorated with what appear to be M& M's (the trademark logo on each piece has been tactfully obscured) and little candy sprinkles.

"From the moment you step into a Marble Slab Creamery, your senses tell you the experience will be anything but ordinary!" screams the ad copy. The ad goes on to describe in salacious detail the sensual richness of both the "super premium" and "reduced-fat" versions of the firm's ice cream—a richness and sensuality that makes Marble Street Creamery an ideal choice "every time you indulge the urge to indulge."

This advertisement is a good example of one of the fastest-growing forms of pornography in America: food porn. The increasing popularity of food porn is probably related to basic demographic trends. As the American population ages, it is discovering, inevitably, that sex is over-rated. Sex fascinates adolescents and strongly interests younger adults.

Baby boomers, as they move into their fifties and beyond, are being re-minded of the fact that food, unlike sex, remains eternally interesting. After all, at any particular time only a minority of the population has anything like an active sex life. Yet everyone, from the baby born this morning to the centenarian who has eaten upwards of one hundred thousand meals, has an extremely active food life.

Human culture has always reflected this truth. Open up the Book of Leviticus, and count the number of divine laws regulating, respec-tively, the kitchen and the bedroom. In this regard, the ancient He-brews merely reflected a universal consensus: In almost all societies, the rules, rituals, and taboos surrounding the provision and consump-tion of food have always been far more numerous, complex, and inter-esting than those surrounding sexuality.

And, now that contraception and a general loosening of societal mores regarding sex have removed much of the savor of what was once forbidden fruit (note the nature of the most common metaphor for erotic transgression), food in America is being overtly charged with quasi-erotic qualities. The idea of a sinful indulgence is now more likely to be associated with an ice-cream cone than with an illicit em-brace; indeed, to utter the very word "fat" has become arguably more transgressive than to use the phrase "semen-stained dress" in polite conversation.

Food taboos are everywhere. It's becoming difficult to hold a din-ner party, or to pick a restaurant, without taking into account food requirements and proscriptions of an almost religious complexity. Be-tween the many varieties of vegetarianism (most notably what chef and author Anthony Bourdain has characterized as "that Hezbollah-like splinter faction, the Vegans"), and the number of "points" each dish will rack up on somebody's Zone or Weight Watchers chart, and the need to provide carbohydrate-free meals for followers of Dr. Atkins or some similar guru, cooking a meal for even a relatively small group can often come to involve negotiations reminiscent of those leading up to the signing of a Middle East peace treaty.

Such negotiations represent the totemic side of our increasingly religious and erotic orientation toward food. The taboo side is re-flected by the menus of high-end restaurants, which often read as if they were written by the same people who churn out the soft-core pornography found within the racier genre of romance novels. Dishes are never cooked: They are "seared," "marinated," and "slowly roasted before your eyes in our open-pit mesquite grill." Foods are "infused" with elaborate herbal extracts, "drizzled" with clarified lemon butter, and "warmed" to a sensual consistency. Contemporary menu prose, so often redolent of a menagerie of gastronomic exotica, can recall a sort of debased version of the reverie in Keats' "The Eve of St. Agnes":

> And still she slept in azure-lidded sleep,
> In blanched linen, smooth, and lavender'd,
> While he from forth the closet brought a heap
> Of candied apple, quince, and plum, and gourd,
> With jellies soother than the creamy curd,
> And lucent syrops, tinct with cinnamon;
> Manna and dates, in argosy transferr'd
> From Fez; and spiced dainties, every one,
> From silken Samarcand to cedar'd Lebanon.

No place better captures our increasingly neurotic orientation toward the totems and taboos of food in America than the average supermarket. The American supermarket, which we enter as if it were the most boring and banal of public spaces, is actually an extraordinary place: a kind of empire of signs, leading us into the contemporary labyrinth that is the American obsession with food, fat, and body image. If we make the effort, we can refocus our eyes, and see the supermarket with something akin to the freshness of an anthropological perspective. By doing so we will find ourselves in a place that is the very opposite of the boring and banal. Indeed, if we visit our local Safeway or Kroger or Piggly Wiggly with just a touch of the anthropologist's openness to the shock of the new, we will soon find ourselves entering into a kind of apocalyptic whorehouse of food lust, and a purifying temple of food abnegation—all within the same fluorescent public space.

The first thing an anthropologically minded visitor to the supermarket will be struck by is the sheer abundance of different things to eat. The aisles seem endless; and each row of tall shelves is packed with immense quantities of food, glorious food. (The economics of the battle for scarce supermarket shelf space is an interesting little story in itself. One would never think that scarcity would be a major issue within a space that contains literally tens of thousands of different food products—but in fact the competition for shelf space is fierce.)

The next thing such a visitor will notice is the staggering variety of foods, and of the subgroups within food groups, and indeed within the same product line. Nine different varieties of Oreo cookies (including reduced fat, of course); twelve types of Lay's potato chips; more than two hundred different kinds of ice cream: Is it any wonder that recent immigrants to the United States, when they first enter a supermarket, are said to sometimes wonder if they have stumbled into some sort of food museum?

The supermarket, it would seem, is a kind of architectural tribute to the cornucopia that is America today, where food is available in greater quantity and variety than in any other culture in the history of the world. Upon closer inspection, however, the story becomes more complicated.

A startling number of the products in this food utopia have been packaged in containers that feature one or more of the following words and phrases: low fat, no fat, fat-free, less fat, light, lite, no cholesterol, lean, non-fat, 50% less fat, 90% fat-free, healthy choice, now with 45% fewer calories, and many, many combinations of, and variations on, these magical signifiers. The visitor to the supermarket is bombarded by hundreds of contradictory messages on every trip down its majestic aisles. Yes, the potential consumer is told, we have an unparalleled selection of food, designed to satisfy every conceivable gastronomic urge. But we, the omniscient gods of consumption, are also well aware of the guilt those urges elicit. Fear not! We will offer you food that is in some fashion less than real food, and yet somehow just as satisfying.

This is the classic logic of diet food advertising: less is more; all the flavor and half the calories; tastes great, less filling. Who says you can't have it all? Well, your taste buds will, the first time you sample a SnackWell's fat-free cookie. (Nabisco's SnackWell's line is currently racking up more than four hundred million dollars in yearly sales in America alone.) Reduced-fat food doesn't taste as good, because fat is one of the things—perhaps the key thing—that makes food taste good. Food that contains fat also tends to satiate hunger much more effectively than low-fat or fat-free food. The statistics are grim: Americans get 20% less of their daily caloric intake from fat than they did a generation ago, yet at the same time ingest 10% more calories per day than they did during more fat-friendly days. We are getting fatter by eating less fat.

The reason is, on one level, extremely simple, and yet somehow almost incredible in a culture that regularly demonizes some aspect of food. (Several critics of the diet industry have pointed out that the current fat phobia has merely displaced—or rather supplemented— earlier bouts of hysteria over sugar, starch, and carbohydrates.) The reason we are getting fatter while eating less fat is that, as Richard Klein points out in his book *Eat Fat*, fat doesn't make people fat—food does.

People feel guilty about eating real food because they think real food makes them fat, which is perceived as a sign of moral weakness, lack of discipline, and, most important, lower class status. Yet anyone who does not embrace the full-on insanity of the most extreme forms of anorexia nervosa must still eat, several times per day, every day. Surveys indicate that dieters (115 million Americans are dieting at any given time) eat fewer regular meals than non-dieters, but snack more often. We are a nation of dieters, and therefore a nation of snackers: The American food industry's own data show that Americans average twenty "food contacts" per day (the French, who eat one of the world's highest-fat diets while remaining markedly slimmer than Americans, average seven).

The marketing genius of consumer capitalism has responded to this situation by providing Americans with an almost endless selection of fat-free and low-fat snack foods. (Marketing research indicates that "fat-free" has replaced "healthy" as the single most desirable phrase in the minds of American food shoppers.) Let's do the math: 115 million dieters times twenty "food contacts" equals, what, 2.3 billion daily opportunities for Americans to make a fat-free, low-fat, light, low cholesterol, healthy choice. And choose they do. Paul Ernsberger points out that some of America's biggest food companies, such as Kellogg's, Campbell's, and Con Agra, who one might think would have a strong incentive to oppose the weight-loss-at-any-cost mentality, actually derive much of their profits from the general hysteria about weight gain: "These companies have extensive lines of diet, or 'lite' or 'low-fat' products," he told me. "Diet foods have much higher profit margins than ordinary foods. Consumers driven by weight anxiety will be willing to spend extra money if they think certain products will help them slim down. Dieters are a gold mine for the food industry, which is interested in creating as many dieters as possible." Ernsberger also points out that, "since women do the most food shopping, they are the main target, and anxious women are highly vulnerable to weight loss claims attached to ordinary food items. Many 'diet' or 'lite' offerings are cheaper to make than their non-diet counterparts, but cost much more."

Indeed, surveys have shown that, when it comes to food choices, a large majority of Americans are strict Manicheans, who believe the gastronomic universe is locked in an eternal struggle between good and evil. According to orthodox dieting theology, some foods are inherently "good," while others are just as ineluctably "bad." The orthodox thus try their best to avoid all contact with "bad" food, by indulging in the innocent (yet still somehow guilty) pleasure of "good" (i.e., fat-free or low-fat, food).

This, it goes without saying, is a prescription for creating binge eaters, which is precisely what tens of millions of American dieters have become. By denying ourselves the food we would prefer to eat, we put ourselves in a position where we must satisfy our cravings with foods that by their nature do not satisfy cravings, and indeed are designed not to do so.

Of all the words of mice and men, the saddest are surely not the following:

> Fifty calories
> In a fat-filled Fig Newton.
> Non-fat? Seventy.

Nevertheless, this dire haiku (which is factually correct: many diet foods actually have more calories than their non-diet counterparts) still captures the essence of a very large source of avoidable human misery. Laura Fraser describes the phenomenon well. Feeling a mid-afternoon urge for something sweet, she "compromises" and buys a box of SnackWell's fat-free (and irony-free) Devil's Food Cookie Cakes:

> Guiltily, as if I were buying pornography, I picked up a box. At home alone, I bit into a cookie. It was chocolately smooth and sweet, then suddenly—it was gone. It had dissolved in my mouth, leaving only a dreary aftertaste. Somehow, I hadn't gotten what I'd been after. I brought the box to the table and had another, and another. The first row of four cookies in the box was gone. Usually I stop after one or two cookies. But not now. I kept wanting satisfaction, thinking I might find it in the next

row. Then there were only four left. They're fat-free, said the
devil on my shoulder. Go ahead.

I had eaten the whole box. I felt miserable, like the woman
in the SnackWell's commercial who attends a Snack Eaters
Anonymous meeting, confessing her sins. "Yesterday I faltered,"
she says, grief-stricken. "I couldn't resist those cookies! I've ru-
ined everything!" She is redeemed and happy at the end of the
ad, however, when she realizes the cookies she ate were fat-
free and couldn't possibly harm her. Unlike me, she didn't read
the label. No fat, to be sure, but 600 calories per box. I could
have had a real meal with dessert instead. And still I didn't feel
satisfied.

As a famous obesity researcher once noted, "the expense of spirit
in a waste of shame is lust in action." And more and more often in
America today, it is a fat-free cookie, rather than some embodiment of
ideal pulchritude, that is "past reason hunted, and no sooner had, past
reason hated."

It isn't an exaggeration to note that, in several crucial respects,
America today is a fundamentally eating-disordered culture. The structure of dieting, which dominates the fashion in which perhaps half of
all Americans relate to food for significant portions of their lives, is the
structure of bingeing and purging, within which the adept seeks a satisfaction no diet food can provide. The cycle of sin and salvation, fall
and redemption, is played out every time the dieter falls off the wagon
(as almost all do), and then climbs back on. The logic behind this pattern is positively Satanic: Dieters gradually rob themselves of all real
pleasure from food, while gradually getting fatter than they ever would
have been if they had just gone ahead and eaten food they actually enjoyed in the first place.

Ironically, as the American palate (at least among the upper classes)
becomes ever more exquisitely hedonized, Americans are eating more
and more pseudo-food that no self-respecting food lover would touch.
Perhaps our food-porn fantasies become ever more elaborate precisely
because so many of us end up settling for a SnackWell's version of food.

Within the temple of sin and redemption that is the American
supermarket, the neurotic and depressing spectacle of food lust collid-
ing with food guilt finds its ultimate expression at the checkout counter.
Here, we who are about to consume are presented with a host of maga-

zines, most of which announce in banner type that, somewhere within their covers, we will find the magic formula that will allow us to eat food without guilt.

What follows is a catalog of magazine teasers visible from one spot at a checkout counter, at a Boulder, Colorado, supermarket, on August 12, 2001:

1. *Glamour*: "Be a Fat-Burning Success Story—Without Starving."
2. *Woman's Day*: "Lose Weight for Good." "Are You a Sugar Addict?"
3. *Good Housekeeping*: "Walk Off 10 lbs—No Dieting!"
4. *Woman's World*: "Lose 4 lbs a Week Eating the Miracle Slimming Food That Melts Off Fat!" "Weight Loss Success—with Prayer."
5. *Prevention* (which advertises itself as "America's #1 Choice for Healthy Living"): "Flatten Your Belly!"
6. *Redbook*: "The Surprising Habit That's Making You Fat."
7. *Cosmopolitan*: "Jaw-Dropping Celeb Diets No One Else Will Tell You."
8. *Fitness*: "15 All-Time Best Weight Loss Secrets: Exclusive Five-Step Plan to Keep It Off." "Firm Up Faster! The Body You Want in 3 Speedy Workouts." "Sleek Sculpted Arms in Seven Easy Moves."
9. *Men's Fitness*: "Shift into Fat-Burning Overdrive Today."
10. *Men's Health*: "Hard Muscles Fast!" "Seven Drinks That Shrink Your Gut."
11. *Men's Workout*: "Ripped Abs! A Great Grid in Two Weeks."
12. *Fit*: "One Great Workout for a Perky Butt, Flat Abs and Thin Thighs."

All these magazines are displayed next to dozens of varieties of candy, chips, and other junk food, perfectly positioned for last-minute impulse buying. Not surprisingly, the content of the stories themselves often deviates from the messages on the magazine covers. The weight loss "secrets" are not secrets, since there are no secrets to weight loss. The quick and speedy workouts to get the body you want are neither quick nor speedy—the authors tend to feel compelled to reveal that, short of surgery, people cannot change the shape of their bodies quickly—nor will they give you the body you want, since the body you have been acculturated to want is not genetically available to at least 99% of the people who want it. (Incidentally almost all these stories reflect the fixation so many Americans have developed with acquiring the perfectly flat belly of a slim sixteen-year-old boy. Indeed, the current fashion craze for low-slung jeans and cropped tops seems to be driven by the fact that, in contemporary America, a suitably exposed band of toned abdominal flesh has become as much of a caste marker as a red dot on an Indian woman's forehead.)

In a less enlightened era, psychologists would perform experiments on dogs, in which the poor creatures would be placed within a maze in which they were forced to make choices that would result in either access to food or an electric shock. The researchers would then randomize the responses that produced either result, so that the dogs could never learn the rules that supposedly governed "good" and "bad" behavior. After a certain time, dogs subjected to this treatment would become so depressed that they would simply lie down and not get up again. In America today human beings are expected to run similar mazes on a daily basis. Of course people get depressed, too—which helps explain why Prozac and its pharmacological cousins are among the nation's most popular drugs. (Indeed, the latest fad among diet doctors is to prescribe an untested combination of Prozac and the diet drug phentermine.)

It would be nice if fitness magazines, diet books, and junk food all came with some sort of seal of approval, similar to that regarding the humane treatment of animals inserted into the credits of many films today: "No people were harmed during the design, production, advertisement, and sale of these products." It would be even nicer if it were true.

5

The King's Two Bodies

THE LEGEND GOES THAT, after hearing Elvis Presley sing, Colonel Tom Parker remarked that he had found a white man who sang like a black man, and that this combination of talents was going to make both Elvis and the Colonel rich. Legend or not, the observation and the prediction both proved to be true enough. Americans have always been fascinated by literal and metaphoric crossings of racial barriers. Toni Morrison's claim that Bill Clinton was America's first black president has a certain ring of truth: There has always been an Elvis-like quality to Clinton—and this quality has been crucial to the charismatic hold the two men continue to exercise over so many of their fellow citizens.

Indeed, Elvis and Bill have many things in common, including the fact that their dietary habits, and the cooks who have catered to them, have long been considered newsworthy topics. We might, for example, wish to ponder the cultural implications of the fact that the *New York Times* carried a lengthy obituary for Mary Jenkins Langston, the woman who cooked for Elvis for many years (she died in June of 2000). The obituary itself is a fascinating document, treating its audience of upper-class readers to a titillating glimpse of the degenerate food rituals of the white trash king of American popular culture.

The obituary cites a BBC documentary entitled *The Burger and the King* (this documentary is evidence that England is one of the few cultures in the world whose obsession with weight approaches America's) that quoted Mrs. Langston on Elvis's eating habits. "He said that the only thing in life he got any enjoyment out of was eating," she said. "And he liked his food real rich." Mrs. Langston, the *Times* notes, cooked the King's meals "in king-sized proportions: cheeseburgers, chicken-fried steaks, hamburger steaks, caramel cakes and family-sized bowls of banana pudding." Clearly, the reader is being taken into a world in which food is consumed in some sort of Dionysian frenzy: a world in which calories are not counted, portions are not weighed, and all manner of dietary perversions take place.

Confronted with the depth of Elvis's depravity, the normally demure *Times* spares its readers none of the horrifying (yet strangely compelling) details. "For breakfast," it quotes Mrs. Langston as saying, "he'd have homemade biscuits fried in butter, sausage patties, four scrambled eggs and sometimes fried bacon. I'd bring the tray up to his room, and he'd say 'This is good, Mary.' He'd have butter running down his arms."

Again, very much in contrast to the *Times'* normally staid style, the obituary's author cannot resist indulging in some ironic humor, at the expense of Mrs. Langston's former employer: "Though legend spread about the scope of Presley's palate, Ms. Langston knew the truth. 'It's not true that Elvis liked burnt bacon sandwiches,' she told the *South Bend Tribune* at an Elvis festival two years ago. 'He liked his bacon very crisp.' "

The obituary climaxes with a description of the genesis of the famed grilled peanut butter and banana sandwiches that will be forever associated with Elvis's name. Mrs. Langston made several unsuccessful attempts to perfect this *pièce de résistance* of Kingly cuisine, before Elvis's father, Vernon, stumbled upon the critical missing step in the creative process: toasting the bread before grilling it. However, "grilling the [toasted] bread to Presley's taste meant using two sticks of butter for every three sandwiches," the *Times* informs its implicitly incredulous readership.

And the *Times* makes sure we do not remain under the misimpression that this veritable sea of butter went to waste. " 'It'd be just floating in butter,' Ms. Langston said at an Elvis commemoration. 'You'd turn it and turn it and turn it until all the butter was soaked up; that's when he liked it.' " After the shock of this final revelation, the obituary concludes rather whimsically, with Mrs. Langston's recipe for Elvis's favorite cornbread. (A photo of Mrs. Langston accompanies the story. The caption reads, "Mary Jenkins Langston, who cooked butter-drenched dishes for Elvis Presley.")

If Alexis de Tocqueville had traveled through contemporary America, he would have told us that those who wish to understand this nation need to understand Elvis Presley—or more precisely the cult of Elvis. And he would have been right. The Elvis cult touches on so many crucial nerves of American popular culture: the ascent of a working-class boy from the most obscure backwater to international fame and fortune; the white man with the soul of black music in his voice; the performer whose music tied together the main strands of American folk music—country, rhythm and blues, and gospel; and, perhaps most compellingly for a weight-obsessed nation, the sexiest man in America's gradual transformation into a fat, sweating parody of his former self, straining the bounds of a jewel-encrusted bodysuit on a Las Vegas stage.

The images of fat Elvis and thin Elvis live together in the popular imagination, like twin brothers struggling for the affection of America's fickle heart. Indeed, when the post office proposed to release a stamp of Presley a few years after his death, it submitted competing designs, each of which reflected the image of one of the King's two bodies. Predictably, perhaps, thin Elvis won out. Yet ultimately, for the hardest core of his fans, many of whom were and are rural and suburban white working-class and lower-middle-class Americans, the fat Elvis of the King's declining years remains closest to their hearts. It is he, trapped within a body that came to represent the transitory nature of youth and beauty, who speaks most eloquently to their own situation, in a country where slimness is so often the prerogative of wealth and privilege.

The fat Elvis also became, in a sense, a blacker Elvis. Because slimness in America tends to correlate with wealth and privilege, it also tends to correlate with whiteness, and especially upper-class whiteness (working-class whites weigh on average about as much as African Americans and Hispanics). Indeed, the sight of fat Elvis can help remind us, once we have become aware of the depth and the extent of the obesity myth in America today, of the ways in which fat prejudice has come to mirror, and even to some extent replace, race prejudice (of course given the demographics of fat and ethnicity, there is considerable overlap between the phenomena).

The most crucial parallel between obesity and race in America is that both concepts are, at the most fundamental biological and medical levels, fictions. Just as there is no biologically valid phenomenon of different races among humans, there is (subject to exceptions at the extreme statistical margin) no medically valid phenomenon of obesity, in the sense of a level of body mass that is in and of itself necessarily unhealthy. In other words, "race" is a phony biological concept in much the same way that "obesity" is a phony disease. Each, of course, is a powerful social construct, and very real in that sense. But the idea that obesity is a disease in the same sense that lung cancer is a disease is just as wrongheaded as is the idea that race is a defining characteristic of discrete sets of humans in the same sense that, for example, blood type is a defining characteristic of discrete sets of humans.

One could say that fat people have a disease in the same sense that Tiger Woods is "black" and Joe Lieberman is "white." That is, Woods is black and Lieberman is white because, and only because, they are defined as being so. A couple of generations ago Lieberman would not have been considered a "white" American in many social contexts; and Woods would not be considered "black" in many cultures today. Indeed Woods has gone out of his way to emphasize that he comes from a blended ethnic and cultural heritage—his mother is Thai—and yet despite this, much of the media continues to refer to him as an African American, period, as if this essentially arbitrary act of definition represented some sort of independently objective "fact." Similarly, "obesity" is a pathological condition in the sense, and only in the sense, that our culture arbitrarily defines certain levels of weight as undesirable. This definition is just as irrational (and just as powerful) as the analogous racial definitions.

Consider the implications of the fact that several studies have found that short men are subjected to various sorts of economic and cultural discrimination, and that "coincidentally" short men suffer from significantly poorer health and higher mortality rates than tall men. One (highly implausible) explanation for the latter fact is that being short is in and of itself a pathological health condition, that is, a disease. A more logical explanation is that the detrimental health effects of being a short man are largely a product of the fact that being a short man is considered undesirable, rather than vice versa. One thing that, rationally speaking, should not affect the relative plausibility of these explanations is whether or not the medical authorities in such cultures have decided that short men are suffering from the disease of "diminutia." (Note, too, that the discovery that tall men tend to live longer than shorter ones has not led to attempts to find ways to make short men tall.)

A belief—even a belief rising to the level of an almost unquestioned social consensus—in the existence of such a "disease" would still not bring the disease into being at the level of biological fact. It is true that, in a sense, the disease would exist—but in the sense that an irrational social construct exists (a sense that, unfortunately, has very real effects). That most people believe the almost infinite variety of human skin tones and other physical features somehow sort themselves out into discrete biological categories called "races" is just as irrational a belief. Race and obesity both illustrate how the social effects of an idea can be very real, even if the idea that produces those effects happens to be false.

Like race, fat has the power to disgust and contaminate. One of the best indications of this power is the extent to which those who seek to avoid contamination will go in their quest to control the burgeoning sense of panic fat elicits. A particularly common method employed to defuse such panic is to make the very idea of being fat—and especially the idea of famous, fashionably thin people becoming fat—a subject of farce. Making fun of things we secretly fear has always been a staple of the broader forms of comedy. Witness the recent phenomenon of fat drag, in which very slim Hollywood stars (a nearly redundant phrase) pretend to be fat, or, more rarely, intentionally become "fat" (i.e., not hyperthin) for performance purposes.

When Robert DeNiro gained 60 pounds to play the role of Jake LaMotta in the 1984 film *Raging Bull*, he won praise for going to what many people considered the most drastic lengths in the pursuit of his craft. Of course DeNiro actually gained this weight in the interests of a more accurate portrayal of his character. By contrast, with one notable exception, the recent fattening of Hollywood stars has been a technological illusion, made possible by the so-called fat suit. According to Tony Gardner, a special-effects expert who has designed several fat suits, the current boom in the cinematic use of fat suits can be traced to the one worn by Eddie Murphy in 1996's *The Nutty Professor* (this film and its sequel *Nutty Professor II—The Klumps* were basically a series of fat jokes. Both were hits). "When [Murphy's character] is running through the city," Gardner says, "and he's in slow motion and you see his body weight shaking and jiggling, you totally buy that that is his physical body. To me, that was the most brilliant use of a fat suit, ever."

Other auteurs seem to have been equally inspired by that sight. In just the past couple of years, Mike Myers has played a grotesquely fat Scotsman in *Austin Powers II*, Martin Lawrence has portrayed a classic "Mammie" figure in *Big Momma's House* (thus combining traditional drag, fat drag, and a kind of quasi-blackface echo of the minstrel show), Martin Short has parodied the talk-show format in *Primetime Glick* (the central organizing principle of the parody is that the host of the show is fat), Julia Roberts has "lost" 60 pounds over the course of *America's Sweethearts*, and Courtney Cox Arquette has worn a fat suit during a teenage flashback sequence on the enormously popular sitcom *Friends*.

Perhaps the most striking recent use of the fat suit has been Gwyneth Paltrow's transformation into a character weighing 350 pounds, in the Farrelly brothers' film *Shallow Hal*. The premise of *Shallow Hal* is particularly interesting. The story revolves around a superficial young man who is always trying to date women who, culturally speaking, are out of his league, that is, models. Eventually he is hypnotized by a self-help guru (in a characteristically postmodern Hollywood touch, the guru is played by actual self-help guru Anthony Robbins) into a mental state in which he only sees women's "inner beauty." Suddenly, he is attracted to "ugly"—this of course means fat—women, most notably Paltrow, who to the rest of the world appears to weigh 350 pounds, but who the main character mistakes for a woman who looks exactly like Gwyneth Paltrow. The film is full of sight gags revolving around the hilariously bizarre idea that a man might find a fat woman attractive (a striptease, a plunge into a swimming pool that rockets a child out of the pool and into a tree, etc.).

Paltrow's own experiences while making the film are revealing. For one thing, wearing a fat suit made her more conscious of how oppressive the current cultural body ideal is. "When people are scrutinizing every angle of your body all the time, it does tend to make you self-conscious. You get super-critical of yourself," she told reporters. "Recently I gained a little weight and, as a result, my butt is a little bigger and people keep commenting on it. [A newspaper] said because of my macrobiotic diet, I was retaining water so my body was no longer as good as it used to be. It's horrible that the film and fashion industry are so fixated on women being thin. If I had naturally been heavier, I'm not certain I would have gotten as far in this industry as I have, and that shocks and disgusts me."

Paltrow's comments also indicate that she recognizes the arbitrariness of the body ideal that has made her a screen icon. "If I had been born in a different era, in Botticelli's day, I would have been considered gross," she says. Nevertheless, she was totally unprepared for what happened to her the first time she donned her fat suit in public: "It was nothing like I thought it was going to be. When I walked through the lobby [of New York's Tribeca Grand Hotel] and while I sat at the bar, no one would make eye contact with me except one waiter. I almost cried I was hurting so much inside. What I realized then, as well as from talking to overweight people, is that people think they are being kind by not looking, but that's the cruelest thing they can do. It makes the person feel so isolated." She adds that her own image as a screen beauty is in large part based on illusion. "My image is based on the photo shoots I've done for magazines. If women are trying to look like those pictures, I want them to know I don't look like that girl either. It's an illusion done with the aid of cameras, makeup and a lot of airbrushing."

The increasing popularity of fat drag in films and television seems to indicate that fat is well on its way to becoming the twenty-first century equivalent of blackface. A recent essay in the *New Yorker* made this very connection, but in a lighthearted fashion that seemed to unintentionally emphasize the extent to which fat hatred has become a kind of psychic replacement for old-fashioned racism: "Filling the space left by blackface, the fat suit is in its golden age, when it can be seen as a cute, sporting transgression against celebrity rather than as a scandalous insult to fat people." It certainly can be seen in that way. That, after all, is exactly the way blackface was seen by the entertainment and media elites in the days of Al Jolson. Black people, needless to say, saw the matter somewhat differently.

In fact, fat drag does fill the precise cultural space once occupied by blackface. When Gwyneth Paltrow dons a fat suit, she is doing something that, within the context of the culture in which she is a movie star, is essentially identical to what movie star Al Jolson did when he blackened his skin. In each case, a celebrity engages in a carnivalesque transgression of perhaps the most crucial social boundary within the celebrity's culture, in order to exploit both the shock value and the comic potential inherent in this sort of boundary breaking.

The effectiveness of such transgressions depends on the existence of a social consensus that there is something inherently funny about a white person pretending to be black, or a thin person pretending to be fat. And what is supposed to be funny about this, in each case, is that such a pretence is always incredible: In a racist society, it is inconceivable that a white person would not want to be white, just as, in a society that fears and loathes fat as much as ours does, it is inconceivable that a thin person would not want to be thin.

The flip side of this consensus is that a racist society will tend to encourage black people to try to become "whiter" than they would otherwise be. Racist ideology will then tend to be reflected in the hierarchy of color within the community of "black" people, with lighter-skinned "blacks" being preferred to darker-skinned individuals. The logical and practical end point of this tendency is reached with the phenomenon of passing, by which a "black" person actually becomes "white."

In America today, it is generally accepted that both overt encouragement to black people to try to become whiter and the phenomenon of passing itself should be considered remnants of a far more racist past. The notion that any mainstream politician or media figure would dare to suggest that it is better to be white than black is highly implausible. Today we recognize that what in Al Jolson's time was considered by a majority of Americans to be a self-evident biological and social truth (that it was better to be white than black) was in fact nothing more than the central organizing principle of the racist ideology of the day.

This basic shift in the culture's attitude toward race is illustrated well by the ambivalent figure of Michael Jackson. Jackson, the self-styled "King of Pop" who consciously strove to equal or supplant the place occupied by Elvis Presley in American culture, went so far as to marry Elvis's daughter: a gesture that almost seemed like some sort of parodic comment on Jackson's own ambiguous identity. I was in Mexico City at the time of their wedding, and the joke making the rounds there—Elvis and Jackson are both enormously popular in

Mexico—was that *el Negro que quiere ser blanca se hay casado con la niña del blanco más negro.* This joke loses a lot in translation, as much of its effect depends on the masculine and feminine forms nouns have in Spanish, but it might be rendered "the black man who wants to be a white woman has married the daughter of the blackest white man."

Part of Jackson's success as a pop icon was no doubt due to the fact that he was a sort of Elvis in reverse—a "black" performer who became increasingly "white" (in his case, quite literally) in ways that were both transgressive and charismatic. Yet while Elvis's metaphorical blackness seemed to cross cultural boundaries in a liberating fashion (although of course it also caused significant controversy, that is, the hip-shaking on the Ed Sullivan show), there has always been something sad, disturbing, and more than a little sinister about Michael Jackson's weird migration toward an almost literal whiteness. It is difficult, in a society that consciously fights against racist thinking, to look at a photograph of Jackson from his days as a teen idol, and then compare it to his gradual metamorphosis as captured in photographs taken ten, fifteen, or twenty years later, without feeling a sense of revulsion against the kind of self-hatred that seems to have impelled his freakish transformation.

And it is at just this point—at the point where one considers the factors that produce this sort of self-hatred—that the analogy between the concepts of "race" and "obesity" becomes particularly instructive. For the analogy breaks down completely when we compare our reaction to Michael Jackson's attempts to achieve whiteness with our reaction to a fat person's attempts to achieve thinness.

Of all the things to which one might object in the orthodox obesity research literature—and there are many candidates to choose from— the single most noxious assertion is that fat people should lose weight because they are discriminated against. This is, in fact, an extremely common claim. Researchers point out (correctly) that fat people face discrimination in employment and housing, that they are considered less desirable marriage partners, and so on. They then use these facts as justifications for recommending dangerous and ineffective "treatments" for the condition that causes this discrimination—treatments that the researchers often all but admit would not be worth the risks involved if fat people were not subjected to such harsh discrimination.

It's difficult to overstate the outrageousness of this argument. Yet as the medical case against obesity continues to fall apart, this claim—

that weight loss should be encouraged because of fat prejudice—is almost inevitably becoming the preferred justification for advising people to lose weight, and for rationalizing the irrationality of the war on fat. Again, it is simply inconceivable that in the United States today we would attempt to "cure" the "disease" of having darker-than-average skin because dark-skinned people still face deeply rooted forms of discrimination (of course it was not that long ago that racial prejudice had just as much eminently respectable scientific and medical backing as fat prejudice has today).

Indeed, the very outrageousness of this argument helps explain why obesity researchers cling so desperately to every scrap of evidence that might bolster the increasingly discredited idea that being of more than average weight is in and of itself a health problem. For once the health rationalization for fat hatred drops away, what are we left with? Nothing more than the very disturbing fact that, in America today, it is better to be thin than fat because fat people are treated worse than thin people. Given our nation's guilty conscience in regard to racial discrimination, it's no wonder that the war on fat is fought with the aid of so much willful blindness.

The relationship between the concepts of race and obesity in America goes beyond parallels and analogies. As we have seen, fat hatred can often serve as a mask for other, often unconscious, forms of prejudice that manifest themselves when observers feel no compunction about expressing the fear and loathing that the sight of fat elicits in them. I said above that the single most noxious assertion in the obesity literature is that fat people should try to become thin as a response to fat prejudice. Actually, this isn't true. The single most noxious line of argument in the literature is that black and Hispanic girls and women need to be "sensitized" to the "fact" that they have inappropriately positive feelings about their bodies.

Readers may suspect that the previous sentence is a bad joke, or at least an exaggeration. I only wish this were so. Several studies have suggested that African-American and Hispanic girls tend to have much more positive body images than white girls. One University of Arizona study found that, while only 10% of the white teenage girls surveyed were happy with their bodies, 70% of the black teenage girls were happy with theirs (the black girls weighed more, on average, than the white girls). When asked to define "beauty," the white girls described their feminine ideal as a woman 5'7" tall, weighing between 100 and

110 pounds (i.e., someone thinner than the average model). By contrast, the black girls described a woman whose body included such features as visible hips and functional thighs. Furthermore, the black girls tended to insist that looking good was more about having "the right attitude" than "the right body." (Is it a coincidence that black women are both far less obsessed with weight than white women, and seem to suffer no significant ill health effects from even extreme levels of fatness? Researchers have been unable to find a relationship between increased mortality and body mass among African-American women who are classified as "morbidly obese.")

Anyway, obesity researchers and diet companies are doing their best to change this unacceptable situation. In recent years, companies such as Weight Watchers and Jenny Craig have targeted much of their advertising specifically toward upwardly mobile black and Hispanic women, since, as Laura Fraser puts it, most white women already "can't make it through a day without getting disgusted with themselves for not having a better—meaning thinner—body." As for obesity researchers, a recent article noted that black girls have better body images and lower rates of eating disorders than white girls, and also noted that they weighed more. "These findings," the authors concluded, "should be used in the development of culturally sensitive Public Health intervention programs to help reduce the high rates of obesity within the black community and encourage black youth to achieve a healthy and reasonable [sic] body size." Here again we see how crucial the health justification remains to all aspects of the war on fat. How would a proposal for "culturally sensitive Public Health intervention programs" sound if it were translated (accurately) as a proposal to make black and Hispanic girls as neurotic about their weight as white girls tend to be, because these groups represent the best opportunity for expanding the market for the useless, expensive, and dangerous products of the weight loss industry? Indeed, once you strip away the phony medical justifications for such proposals, they end up sounding about as appetizing as a peanut butter and banana sandwich fried in three sticks of butter must sound to the average reader of the *New York Times*.

6

The Bimbo Culture

IT'S A SCORCHING SUMMER DAY, and I'm trapped in my rental car, driving aimlessly around west Los Angeles. I'm looking for the track on the UCLA campus. My goal this morning is to run ten thousand meters in less than forty-six minutes. I've come to Los Angeles for a wedding, and I don't want to pass up the opportunity to try to set a new "PR" (personal record) at sea level.

It doesn't take too much wandering through its streets to be reminded that Westwood—the fashionable section of the city between Beverly Hills and Bel Air that houses UCLA's campus—is just about Ground Zero in America's constantly intensifying war on fat. The ads for weight loss products are everywhere—on billboards, on buses, on the car's radio. "Lose 40 pounds in a month!" one promises (this would seem to require amputating a limb, which for all I know may be the latest innovation in weight loss surgery).

I finally find the track, and end up circling it twenty-five times in a somewhat disappointing forty-six minutes forty-eight seconds (I had been hoping to break forty-six minutes). During the course of the time trial, I lap a pair of college-age women several times. In most cultures they would be considered disturbingly thin. Here, they might be defined as "a little chunkier than your average young actress." They are jogging very slowly; given their appearance they may well be weak from hunger.

I drive back to my hotel in the downtown district, where the streets are full of Mexicans and Central Americans. A lot of them are fat. Nobody is fat in Westwood, except for the hired help. I turn on the television. Jake of *Body by Jake*, the personal trainer to the stars, is selling a "bun and thigh rocker." Fascinated, I watch several minutes of the infomercial, in which Jake tells us that we can eliminate the "flaws" in our "problem areas" in just three minutes a day, without breaking a sweat. He guarantees that, if we call now, we will lose a full dress size in ten days, or our money back. The infomercial is packed with testimonials from people who lost seven pounds and two inches in ten days. The pitch is that you can get into "great" (this of course means thin) shape immediately, by simply rocking back and forth on Jake's contraption.

The problem areas to which Jake refers are the thighs, hips, and butt. Studies indicate that, when women are asked to estimate the dimensions of their hips and thighs, they overestimate by about 20%. Jake is doing his best to raise that number. Not coincidentally the "problem areas" on women's bodies are the areas that make them look like women. (Interestingly, some of the studies that indicate women consistently overestimate their actual body size also suggest men prefer women to weigh, on average, about 20 pounds more than women think men prefer them to weigh.)

Where, I wonder, are the mainstream feminist organizations on this issue? When is the last time NOW or the like had something to say about the fact that a significant portion of the nation's economy is based on making women feel as if they must do everything possible to acquire the bodies of teenage boys? With this thought I find that I've had enough of Jake. I flip over to CNN, where they're talking about Gary Condit. We see video of Condit fleeing the press. The big news today is that Condit has agreed to do an interview with Connie Chung. Chung wears a size 4 (maybe 6) dress, so we know she must be a top-notch reporter. Suddenly, I realize the truth about Gary Condit, which in a certain sense is the truth about America today.

Gary Condit is a preacher's son from the middle of nowhere, who had never accomplished anything notable prior to getting elected, at the age of thirty-four, to the California State Assembly. Condit wasn't a war hero or a successful businessman. He didn't invent a better mousetrap or rise within the ranks of an important public or private institution. He didn't even achieve academic distinction: the last refuge of those who have no other claim to fame on their resumes. He was basically a salesman who went into politics because he looked good on television and could memorize a list of talking points without stumbling over too many of them. Condit succeeded in politics in large part because he was tall and thin, had good hair, "craggy" good looks, and a certain degree of charm. He is, in a word, a bimbo. And that's when it hits me: We are living in a bimbo culture.

Of course in many fields appearance has always counted for a great deal. We have long taken it for granted that models and film stars are supposed to literally embody the reigning cultural ideal of beauty, whatever it happens to be. What has changed is the sheer number of fields in which appearance has come to be considered an important— and often the most important—attribute. In journalism, business, politics, art, sports, and academia it may not be the case that image, as Andre Agassi once put it, is everything, but it's increasingly coming to seem that way.

Consider Agassi's own sport of tennis. A dozen years ago, Agassi was already the world's highest-paid tennis player, even though he hadn't won any of the sport's major tournaments. He was handsome, charming, and talented, and that was enough. That he went on several years later to actually become a great player was almost incidental. An even more striking example is the case of Anna Kournikova, who has made tens of millions of dollars in endorsements, even though she has never won a professional tournament of any kind. In the summer of 2000 *Sports Illustrated* did an eight-page pictorial spread on Kournikova. This was in the same month that the less photogenic Lindsey Davenport won Wimbledon, the sport's most important tournament (Davenport's victory was given scant textual and almost no photographic recognition by the magazine, leading one to wonder what sports, exactly, they are illustrating).

Indeed, sports are often a good marker of changing cultural trends. A generation ago, the slim and handsome Arnold Palmer was crowned the king of the golf world, even though the burly Jack Nicklaus beat him consistently. Nicklaus was nicknamed "Fat Jack" by reporters—a name that stuck with him until, bowing to the growing cultural pressure to be thin, he shed 40 pounds at the height of his career. Today, Tiger Woods dominates golf as thoroughly as Jack Nicklaus dominated the game in the 1960s. A fat Tiger Woods might well be every bit as good a golfer (losing weight did not improve Nicklaus's already peerless game), but he certainly would not be the cultural icon he has become. Sponsors are not going to pay a fat golfer forty million dollars per year to endorse their products, no matter how many tournaments he might win.

In recent years journalism, and television journalism in particular, has come to value image over substance to a remarkable degree. Ed Murrow would never be given a news show to host today: His Q rating simply wouldn't be high enough. Murrow might still do the behind-the-scenes reporting, but his words (suitably edited to take into account the sensitivities of key advertisers) would be put in the mouths of the likes of Deborah Norville and Stone Phillips. Recently, the comedy program *Saturday Night Live* did an amusing sketch, in which an actor playing the role of Phillips did numerous takes of links introducing segments of *Dateline NBC*. ("Next, we have a report on dangerous children's toys," etc.) The sketch was funny because of its pointed emphasis that journalists like Phillips don't really *do* anything: They just stand there looking good, while introducing the work others have done. In other words, they are models. And yet these journalistic mannequins are considered the stars of their profession, and are paid accordingly. The portrayal of the William Hurt character in the film *Broadcast News*—the clueless news anchor who is fed "content" through an earpiece—which even as recently as a decade ago still had some flavor of satire, would today appear almost documentary-like.

The business world also seems to have been overrun by Princeton MBAs with good hair and nice teeth. Since so much of our economy revolves around selling people things that will supposedly make them look good, it stands to reason that the people who are directing the firms that are creating this demand should look the part. The glossy money magazines to which Greg Critser's anti-fat essay referred are filled with flattering portraits, in both senses of the word, of captains of industry and bold entrepreneurs who haven't invented anything or otherwise visibly increased the wealth of the world. Many a contemporary titan of business has, in the wake of the end of the bull market of the 1990s, been exposed as a well-dressed idiot, whose talent turned out to be the ability to look good while uttering clichés on *Wall Street Week* and *The Nightly Business Report*.

Again, television comedy captures the essence of the trend: An episode of *The Simpsons* revolves around Homer's acquisition of hair from a miracle hair-restoring tonic. Suddenly the formerly bald oaf becomes a respected business leader, whose (ghostwritten) speeches are lapped up by his audience. The effect of the tonic wears off in the middle of a speech, causing his hair to fall out all at once, and leading his listeners to start asking "who's that bald man up there, and what are those ridiculous things he's saying?" (The flip side of all this is that the cliché of the techie nerd—the software genius who weighs 275 pounds and wears a pocket protector—captures the general suspicion that when people really need to know how to fix what's broken, it's probably best not to discriminate too much on the basis of appearance.)

Even in the literary world, where a writer's text has traditionally interposed itself between the writer's audience and his dust jacket photo (if any), appearance is coming to play a larger and larger role. Short stories published in high-profile magazines now routinely include fetching photographs of their authors; and literary critics have noted that the new writers whose work is most heavily promoted by prominent presses are beginning to look more like potential GQ and Vogue cover subjects than the next J.D. Salinger.

Anyone involved in academia can attest to the nontrivial effects that appearance and self-presentation can have on the evaluation of ideas. At the typical American university an Oxbridgian accent is generally worth around twenty IQ points. (At one especially prestigious institution located in central New Jersey, the premium put on a fancy accent is so high that people who grew up in Shaker Heights, Ohio, often sound as if they spent their formative years in Prague cafés, arguing about the destiny of Central Europe with Vaclav Havel.) Other classic examples of the effect of appearance on the reception of ideas can be found in the history of contemporary feminism, which includes such events as the author of *The Feminine Mystique* being supplanted as a leading national feminist figure by a former Playboy bunny.

But it is in the world of politics that the bimbo culture is having some of its most striking and invidious effects. Consider the 2000 presidential election. Many people noted that George W. Bush could never have been elected president if he were not the son of George Herbert Walker Bush. And of course it remains a truism of American politics that only white men are, at present, eligible to become major presidential candidates. Yet what went generally unnoted was that the younger Bush could not have been elected if he had happened to be fat or bald or short. Al Gore, too, was the recipient of the advantages that go with being born into a powerful political family. Yet his campaign advisers emphasized to him that he needed to lose 30 pounds before the campaign got under way, which he duly did (predictably, he has since regained the lost weight).

Gore's advisers had seen what happened to Bill Clinton when Clinton gained weight over the course of the 1992 presidential campaign. And, as we shall see, even though Clinton only became "fat" in the eyes of those who are so obsessed with weight issues that, for them, everyone who is not unnaturally thin is by definition fat, Clinton's supposed fatness became the focus of so many jokes that those around him (including, most significantly, Hillary Clinton) took aggressive steps to slim him down to a more "presidential" weight—steps that ended up playing a key role in triggering the series of events that led to Clinton's impeachment.

Perhaps the most revealing aspect of the 2000 election was the choice of running mates for Bush and Gore. Dick Cheney and Joe Lieberman were universally acclaimed to be superior candidates to the men at the top of the ticket. Cheney, in particular, continues to be seen as the brains behind the pretty boy façade provided by W. himself. Bald and heavyset, Cheney simply does not have an appropriate body for a contemporary presidential candidate. Lieberman is fashionably thin, but as a balding Jewish man he seems doubly disqualified from occupying the Oval Office.

It is a remarkable fact of American life that, even as the idea of someone like Hillary Clinton or Colin Powell as president is becoming thinkable, the appearance standards for politicians in terms of purely cosmetic issues such as weight are becoming increasingly restrictive. In short, what might be labeled the Gary Condit Phenomenon represents the essence of the bimbo culture. Basically, it appears that more and more people in America today are in positions of power and influence because they have what the culture considers an appropriate physique. And while the standards for factors such as height, ethnicity, and even gender display a certain degree of flexibility, the standards surrounding fat do not. (While it is certainly possible to imagine George Stephanopoulos becoming president, it is not possible to imagine Madeline Albright ascending to that office—and not primarily because she is a woman.)

What American culture considers appropriate is a body that signals its owner is in control of that body's desires. This, fundamentally, is the metaphorical significance of thinness in America today. In other words, Americans—and especially American elites—value thinness for precisely the same reason someone suffering from anorexia nervosa does: because not eating means not giving in to desire. Strangely, what the American elites consider most desirable is a body whose appearance signals a triumph of the will over desire itself. Thus, bodily virtue is not so much indicated by thinness per se, but rather by an *achieved* thinness.

In contemporary America, the truly virtuous soul is found within the fat person who inhabits a thin body. This helps explain why the cultural ideal in terms of body weight is being ratcheted constantly downward. Even under present cultural conditions, where the combination of lots of cheap, good-tasting food and an increasingly sedentary lifestyle makes it easy to put on weight, many women of average height can still weigh 135 pounds without dedicating a good portion of their lives to achieving and maintaining that weight. But what virtue is there in that? The average 5'4" woman who weighs 115 pounds, on the other hand, can rarely maintain that weight without suppressing many of her most powerful (and healthy) desires at every turn. Those are the "extra" 20 pounds that millions of American women (and, increasingly, men) are so desperate to shed: 20 pounds that have nothing to do with health—indeed, all other things being equal, it is probably healthier for an average-height woman to weigh 135 rather than 115 pounds—and everything to do with the need to conform to an oppressive, irrational, and unjust ideal.

Consider three women of average height, each of whom weighs 115 pounds. Anna eats normally—that is, she neither diets nor binges—while consuming an average of 2,200 calories per day of well-balanced nutrition. She is moderately active. Maya diets rigorously; she makes sure not to consume more than 1,500 calories per day; she avoids all high-fat and high-sugar foods; and she exercises intensely for at least ninety minutes six times per week. Zoe consumes an average of 2,700 calories per day, much of it in the form of junk food. She is almost completely sedentary.

There is nothing unusual about these hypothetical examples: As we shall see, normal variations in human physiology ensure that people who consume very different numbers of calories and engage in widely varying degrees of activity can end up with exactly the same body mass. Such variations also ensure that people who eat the same number of calories, and are similarly active, will nevertheless end up at far different weight levels.

The obesity myth is built around the false belief that it is possible to determine whether someone has a healthy lifestyle by observing whether that person maintains a "healthy" [sic] weight. Of course Anna, Maya, and Zoe are all given powerful cultural incentives to accept this myth. Anna, who actually does have a healthy lifestyle, would naturally like to believe that her "healthy" weight reflects this fact. Maya, whose life is organized around maintaining a regimen of disordered eating and compulsive exercising, has an even stronger incentive to believe that the extraordinary—and in the long run almost surely unsustainable—efforts she is making to maintain a weight significantly below what she would maintain if she ate normally and exercised moderately are justified by health concerns. As for Zoe, she lives in a culture that believes the shape of her body proves she has a disciplined and virtuous approach to food and exercise: an irrational belief that she may well share, and that in any case she has no incentive to dispel.

In other words, the cultural politics of fat cause millions of Americans to imbue an extremely narrow range of weight—a range that is far narrower than that which actually occurs among people who live healthy lives—with a medical and moral significance it does not have. To acknowledge the truth that healthy people come in all shapes and sizes, and that many people maintain so-called ideal weight levels despite unhealthy lifestyles, would rob thinness of its virtue-conferring power.

The bimbo culture advertises itself as a celebration of youth, beauty, and sexiness. In the end, it has very little to do with any of those things. Rather, our current obsession with maintaining an absurdly thin body has more to do with darker strains in the American character—with that part of American culture that has always distrusted desire in general, and has now come to fear food in particular, as a harbinger of sloth, gluttony, lust, and every other deadly consequence of uncontrolled indulgence in life's pleasures.

Our hyperthin celebrities, whether they are entertainers or politicians—a distinction that has become increasingly meaningless—present us with images of virtuous denial: "I do not eat, therefore I am (famous)." Someone like Madonna, who is said to work out for several hours every day, and who for a time entered every bite of food that went into her mouth into a computer program, could be considered a sort of secular saint of this culture: a kind of unholy anorexic, denying herself food so that we might live out our fantasies of unlimited indulgence through her.

Madonna, and those like her—roughly speaking, *People* magazine's A-list—are not so much singers or actors or journalists or politicians as they are hunger artists. For as we shall see, in the end the bimbo culture is essentially the culture of anorexia nervosa.

7

Weight Problems

ALTHOUGH OBESITY has not yet been criminalized in the United States, it's possible to have your three-year-old child taken from you for the offense of "allowing" her to become fat. That is the stark lesson of the Anamarie Regino saga, which continues to play out in Albuquerque, New Mexico. The story of what was done to a child and her parents by an assortment of doctors, social workers, and government bureaucrats is a chilling tale of what can happen when people of modest means and social status find themselves, through no fault of their own, facing the full brunt of the prejudice that fuels the war on fat.

Anamarie—who weighed 6 pounds, 13 ounces at birth—gained 32 pounds in her first eight months of life. Her mother, Adela Martinez-Regino, realized from the beginning that there was something different about her daughter. "She was drinking ten and twelve bottles a day and still wanting more, " she says. So Martinez-Regino, a native New Mexican and a counter agent for Mesa Airlines, started taking her daughter to doctors, in what became an increasingly desperate attempt to determine why her daughter was so large. (Besides her weight, Anamarie soon grew to be nearly twice as tall as other children her age, and developed a full set of teeth by the time she was a year old.)

Over the next few months, a parade of pediatricians, endocrinologists, and specialists in rare childhood syndromes examined Anamarie.

None of them was able to successfully diagnose her condition. By the time the girl was sixteen months old, her mother had taken Anamarie to fifty-seven doctors' appointments, yet her condition remained as mysterious as ever. And still, Anamarie continued to grow at a remarkable rate: She weighed 67 pounds at sixteen months, 97 pounds at twenty-eight months, and 130 pounds by July of 2000, when she was a little more than three years old.

The following month, after Anamarie's parents hospitalized her for a third time in an Albuquerque hospital for yet more tests, her mother was taken aside by a group of doctors and social workers. In Martinez-Regino's words, she was told "Ana's in grave danger. We know it's hard to say no to a three-year-old. We know it's hard not to give in to everything she wants. We just think you can't handle your daughter. And we don't want her to die down the line."

What Anamarie's mother didn't know was that the state's Child, Youth and Families Department was already preparing an affidavit that would accuse her and her husband, Miguel Regino, of endangering their child's life by making her fat. According to the social workers who filed this document, Anamarie would "surely die" if she was not placed immediately on a rigid diet and exercise program. This, the social workers said, was "something which the parents have not been willing or able to do." The affidavit concluded with some devastating charges. New Mexico's social service bureaucracy claimed that Anamarie's "family does not fully understand the threat to their daughter's safety and welfare due to language or cultural barriers." Furthermore, the social workers said, Anamarie might be a victim of Munchausen's syndrome by proxy—a psychological disorder that causes parents to harm their children in order to draw attention to themselves.

The next few days were a nightmare for Anamarie's parents. They were told the hospital would call security if they tried to take their child home. Deeply confused and angered by the charges being made against them, they watched with a growing sense of helplessness as the state proceeded to take Anamarie from them. Martinez-Regino's description of the final scene would chill the blood of any parent. On the morning of August 25, they were forced to explain to their three-year-old that "you will be going to stay with some different people now, but Mommy and Daddy will come to visit." Her mother recalls that, as a nurse pushed the child away down the hospital hall in a stroller "she kept screaming that she wanted her daddy to push her. But we knew there were armed guards outside, so we couldn't do anything. It was so difficult to sit there and do nothing because you could hear her scream all the way down the hall."

It's difficult to describe the sheer irrationality of the decision process that led to this appalling abuse of state power. Here are just some of the aspects of this fiasco that illustrate the depths of the craziness to which the war on fat can drive public officials:

➤ At the time she was taken into state custody, there was no evidence that Anamarie's health was in danger. Despite her extraordinary size, an almost endless battery of tests had concluded that she was not suffering from any detectable cardiovascular problem, or any other major medical difficulties. Despite this, the state social workers' affidavit claimed that Anamarie was in grave danger of suffering "fatal heart damage" if she was not taken from her parents immediately.

➤ Although the justification for taking Anamarie from her parents was that she was in immediate medical danger, the state took her from the hospital into which her parents had admitted her three times in the previous few weeks, and moved her to a private foster home, where she remained for the next two and a half months.

➤ The state's affidavit charged Anamarie's parents with being unable or unwilling to keep the child on an appropriate diet, when in fact they had, on the advice of a constantly shifting cast of health-care experts, placed her on a series of diets, all of which they followed faithfully. These diets began at 1,200 calories per day, then declined to 1,000 calories, then 900, and finally 550. This final diet, which Anamarie was on at the time she was taken from her parents, consisted of two Kindercal drinks (two such drinks might make up perhaps a third of a normal three-year-old's daily caloric intake). In other words, Anamarie's parents were being told to starve their child—yet even after agreeing to do so they were accused of causing, or at least seriously exacerbating, her still-mysterious condition, by feeding her "too much."

That there could even be a discussion about whether the state ought to take a child away from her parents under these circumstances indicates how severely the topic of fat distorts public debate in America today. It should be unnecessary to point out that the whole idea that parental dietary practices might play a significant role in producing a 130-pound three-year-old is absurd. Such a theory is every bit as bizarre as the idea that Anamarie's parents were damaging her health by forcing her to become twice as tall as other children her age. Anyone who has ever parented small children knows how difficult it is to get them to eat something they would prefer not to eat. As for "overfeeding" a toddler, lax parental supervision of a toddler's eating habits might result in a three-year-old weighing five or perhaps even ten pounds more than she would otherwise weigh—but at the time of her third hospitalization Anamarie weighed 90 pounds more than the average three-year-old.

Anamarie's mother is not an obesity expert, but she is perfectly capable of critiquing the bizarre idea that her daughter is three times heavier than a normal toddler because her parents have made her that way. "If we are overfeeding her, then why is she so tall?" Martinez-Regino asks. "Why did she have all her teeth by the time she was a year old? Why does she have thick hair, adult kind of hair? Can overfeeding do all that?" Martinez-Regino is also well aware of the subtext of the state's claim that Anamarie's family "does not understand the threat to their daughter's safety and welfare due to language and cultural barriers." A working-class woman of Mexican heritage living in Albuquerque, married to a man who does not speak English well, doesn't need a doctorate in sociology to understand the threat to her parental rights emanating from that sentence. When she read those words in the affidavit, Martinez-Regino says, "I knew they decided about us before they even spoke to us."

Leslie Prichard, a paralegal and the wife of Anamarie's parents' lawyer, Troy Prichard (the Prichards took on the case for free) asks the obvious question: If her parents had been white, upper-class professionals, would they have been charged with child abuse simply because their daughter was unusually large? Troy Prichard has little doubt about what led the state to take such drastic action. "There were so many veiled comments which added up to 'You know those Mexican people, all they eat is fried junk, of course they're slipping her food.' That's what they wanted to see."

Yet whatever part class and ethnic prejudice may have played in the decision to take Anamarie from her parents, it seems clear that another factor played an even bigger role. "Everybody we were dealing with was skinny. There were no overweight doctors," said Martinez-Regino. "People sometimes look at her and think she sits in front of the TV and eats and eats. But ever since she was a baby she's been moving around . . . It comes down to some people are fat because they have a condition. But the public, they don't look at it as a medical problem. They look at it as a mental problem. Her weight will go up and down. She will never be a Barbie."

Anamarie's story has a happy ending, at least to this point. Two and a half months after she was taken from her parents, Troy Prichard negotiated an agreement whereby the state retained legal custody of Anamarie pending a hearing. In exchange, her parents regained physical custody of their child. For the next two months Anamarie lived at her parents' modest cinderblock house again, while a cadre of social workers made regular visits, during which they sat on the family's living room couch and observed her interactions with her parents. As part of the agreement Martinez-Regino agreed to be evaluated by a psychiatrist, who found no evidence of Munchausen's syndrome by proxy or any related psychological problems. In January 2001, a New Mexico state judge dismissed the charges of child abuse the state had filed against her parents, and returned legal custody of Anamarie to them.

Since then Anamarie has become something of a celebrity in the battle against fat prejudice. In a particularly galling irony, her parents have been accused of exploiting her situation to gain media attention. Such charges ignore the fact that Adela Martinez-Regino and Miguel Regino never sought to be accused of child abuse by the state of New Mexico, and that, given the underlying cultural politics of their situation, fighting the battle to win back their child through the media was one of their few realistic options. To this day, Anamarie's parents realize they are under more or less constant surveillance whenever they take their daughter outside their home. Recently a state social worker called them to let them know the department had received a report that Anamarie had been seen eating ice cream. Her mother was forced to explain to the authorities that her child had been eating frozen yogurt—an approved treat within the strict confines of Anamarie's latest diet, which forbids all candy, cake, ice cream, juice, fried food, or fast food.

As of this writing, Anamarie weighs 105 pounds—approximately

25 pounds less than she did at her heaviest. In addition to her strictly monitored diet, she spends three days per week at a local gym for children, called Kid Power. Here she swims, jumps, and exercises muscles that have to be much stronger than an average child's to simply allow her to walk.

Troy and Leslie Prichard are preparing a civil suit against many of the doctors and social workers involved in the decision to take Anamarie from her parents. Ironically, her parents plan to use any proceeds from this suit to take their child to "the best doctors in America," who they still believe will be able to determine why their daughter is the way she is, and to give her condition a name. For Anamarie's family, this last desire is not a minor point. Her godmother, says Martinez-Regino, is planning to have cards printed for the benefit of inquiring strangers, who still insist on asking questions about "what is wrong" with their daughter, and, of course, about what her parents feed her. "The cards," says Anamarie's mother, "will give the name of the condition and explain what it is. Then they'll say, 'Now mind your own business!' "

The story of Anamarie Regino tells us a great deal about the meaning of fat in America today. It tells us that, for all its pretensions to knowledge, the medical profession still understands very little about the causes and consequences of much of what is labeled "obesity." No one has been able to determine why Anamarie's body is the way it is. Furthermore, no one knows if her size endangers her health (how could anyone know this, given the complete failure to diagnose the nature of the underlying condition?). It follows that no one knows whether it's in Anamarie's best interests to severely limit her diet. That a barely three-year-old child was put on a starvation diet of 500 calories per day says nothing about the potential efficacy of such a radical treatment (again, as is so often the case with weight issues and medicine, the Hippocratic injunction to "first do no harm" was ignored in Anamarie's case), but it does say a great deal about the hysteria that fat elicits among so many doctors, social workers, and other members of the helping professions.

Anamarie's story also illustrates the strength of the American belief that a person's weight is something that is fundamentally under his or her control, or, in the case of small children, under the control of their parents. This belief is so deeply entrenched that it manifests itself in situations in which it can only be described as profoundly irrational. Perhaps the only thing that frightens Americans more than the thought of getting fat is the thought that there is often, practically speaking, little or nothing people can do about getting fat. One explanation for the absurdity of the state's response to Anamarie's situation is that her skyrocketing weight became a kind of metaphor for the anxiety so many Americans feel about their (or their spouse's, or children's, or fellow citizens') expanding waistlines.

Most alarmingly, Anamarie's saga helps reveal the lengths to which state power can be deployed in America today in the prosecution of the war on fat. Adela Martinez-Regino and Miguel Regino cannot allow their child to eat a spoonful of ice cream, or a piece of candy, or to drink a glass of fruit juice, without running a very real risk of having their child taken away from them once again. They and Ana live under this remarkably repressive regimen not because there is any medical evidence that it will protect their daughter's health, but simply because it gives the authorities a false but comforting sense that they are "doing something" about what is, for them, a profoundly disturbing sight—the sight of an unusually large child.

The same social hysteria that inspired Greg Critser's apocalyptic essay on the meaning of fat in America manifested itself in Anamarie's case, but with far graver results than the publication of a poorly researched magazine article. And, as was the case with Critser's essay, Anamarie's story illustrates the intimate relationship between, on the one hand, slenderness and power, privilege, and money, and, on the other, fat and powerlessness, lack of social status, and relative poverty. In both instances, these dichotomies manifested themselves along ethnic lines as well. (The Hispanic social worker who interviewed Martinez-Regino when the state began the process of taking her child from her insisted on doing so in Spanish, despite the fact that English is Martinez-Regino's first language. According to Martinez-Regino, the social worker kept demanding the telephone numbers of her family in Mexico, even though Martinez-Regino was born in the United States and has spent her entire life here.)

Perhaps the most striking irony of Anamarie's story is the faith her family maintains in doctors and medicine. Despite being accused by doctors, on the basis of no evidence whatsoever, of abusing their child, Anamarie's parents cling to the belief that doctors can be trusted to explain the meaning of what has happened to their daughter. Ultimately, it is this faith—a very American faith in the ability of science and technology to answer what are, in the most fundamental sense, political and cultural, rather than scientific, questions—that plays perhaps the most crucial role in supporting the war on fat.

What remains difficult to see, even for those who have paid the heaviest price in that war, is that it isn't people like Anamarie who have a weight problem. We live in a nation in which those in authority can look at a three-year-old girl with the "wrong" sort of body and decide, on the basis of nothing more than irrational beliefs born of their own fear and loathing of fat, that her family must be torn apart. Now *that* is a weight problem.

8

All the News That's Print to Fit

A N OLD JOURNALISTIC APHORISM asserts that in war, truth is the first casualty. The war against fat illustrates this point particularly well. One of the keys to that war is the success with which the weight loss industry has managed to spread its propaganda through the nation's media. Journalists routinely reprint self-serving interpretations of data provided to them by obesity researchers—researchers whose work is often funded by firms that have an overwhelming economic interest in the proposition that "obesity" is a major health risk. That the economic structure of obesity research is so heavily skewed toward a desire to conclude that fat kills does not, by itself, discredit that conclusion. But one would hope it would cause journalists to approach that conclusion with the sort of skepticism the situation warrants. This they have in large part failed to do.

Ideally, when reporting on the relationship between weight and health, journalists would take into account that obesity research has been particularly prone to the various forms of statistical manipulation outlined in the first part of this book. They would also be aware that the available evidence regarding the relative risks of overweight, underweight, weight gain, and weight loss does not support the weight loss industry's and the public health establishment's contention that a BMI of 25 or higher ought to be considered a significant independent health risk. Journalists covering this issue would be expected to know that numerous studies have indicated that physical activity levels are far better predictors of health and mortality than body mass, and they would ask hard questions of researchers who made claims on the basis of studies that failed to control for these factors. They would also know something about the extensive literature that has found associations between dieting and increased mortality, and they would be aware that studies have identified social discrimination as a significant negative factor in regard to both maintaining good health and having access to health care. In short, they would question the assumption at the heart of the war on fat that weight loss (rather than lifestyle changes that usually have little or no effect on weight) is the key to improving the health of the American public.

Unfortunately, in modern American journalism, even the best regarded media sources have proven quite unreliable when the story has involved the supposed health dangers of "excess" weight. What follows is a typical example of how the issue of the relationship between weight and health gets distorted by reporting that fails to ask the hard questions that, at this point, should be a standard part of any good journalist's investigation of America's obsession with weight and weight loss.

The *Wall Street Journal* is one of the world's great newspapers. Many journalists will tell you that it features perhaps the best staff of reporters of any paper in America. In other words, if a story isn't being reported accurately in the *Journal*, chances are it isn't being reported accurately in any mainstream media source.

Given this, consider the implications of the following piece of reportage, taken from the August 9, 2001, edition of the paper. The *Journal*'s "What's News" feature, running down the length of the second and third columns on the front page, contains the following item: "Diabetes researchers have found that medication or a combination of diet and exercise can prevent the adult-onset form of the disease, which is most common. Weight loss is the best defense. (Article on Page B1)." For the *Journal*'s two million or so daily readers, this abstract will be crucial to whatever understanding they take away from the article. Most will probably not read the article itself; many that do will only skim it.

Those who do turn to the story will encounter the following lead paragraph, which I quote in its entirety: "Losing just a modest amount of weight can cut the risk of developing type 2 diabetes in half for people who are at high risk for the disease, according to a new large-scale study."

It seems certain that almost all of the *Journal's* readers who encounter the front-page abstract and the story's opening paragraph will come away with the idea that the key to fighting adult-onset diabetes is to lose weight. Only those who bother to read the story carefully, and with a critical eye, will ever notice that the study indicated almost exactly the opposite of what the *Wall Street Journal* said it did.

Here are the facts: The study followed more than three thousand volunteers for at least three years. The volunteers had an average BMI of 34, which translates into a weight of 197 pounds for an average-height woman (5'4") and 236 pounds for an average-height man (5'10"). The volunteers adopted a low-fat diet, and started exercising thirty minutes per day, several days per week. After three years, the average volunteer had lost a total of 8 pounds (i.e., a trivial percentage of body mass for persons that began the study weighing, on average, around 220 pounds). Yet the volunteers cut their risk of developing diabetes by 58%. (A trial of the drug Glucophage, conducted simultaneously, found it was roughly half as effective in preventing diabetes, in comparison to the benefit gained from these changes in diet and exercise.)

The story quotes David Nathan, the study's chairman, as being surprised that changes in lifestyle could have such beneficial effects. In fact, this should not have surprised those who have followed the by now extensive literature on the health benefits of good nutrition and exercise, which have been shown to have similarly beneficial effects on high blood pressure, cholesterol levels, and other medical risk factors, without regard to whether these lifestyle changes lead to any weight loss. For example, previous studies of the effects of lifestyle changes carried out by Finnish and Japanese researchers had already shown similar success in fighting adult-onset diabetes. This new study confirmed and broadened those earlier findings, by testing a more ethnically diverse population (45% of the volunteers came from ethnic groups—in particular African Americans and Hispanics—whose members seem especially prone to developing diabetes).

The *Wall Street Journal's* coverage of this story is typical of the coverage of weight-related health issues in the United States. Actually, unlike most of the stories regarding it in other newspapers, the *Journal's* summary of the study was at least statistically accurate. Most media outlets reported that the volunteers had lost an average of about

15 pounds, when in fact after an initial weight loss of slightly less than that, most of the subjects began to gain weight again. The confusion seems to have arisen because the study's authors had said their initial goal was to get volunteers to lose at least 15 pounds; typically, soon after this modest weight loss goal was achieved, the average volunteer regained much or all of the lost weight. These complicating details, which when taken together more or less destroy the "lose weight to avoid diabetes" storyline, were left out of almost all of the other media reports.

Even the *Journal,* which reported the data from the survey accurately, used examples from the data pool that were potentially quite distorting. For instance, of the two volunteers the paper interviewed, one's weight was not reported, while the other's weight had reduced from 214 to 183 pounds over the course of the study. This represents a degree of weight loss almost 400% greater than the average amount of weight lost by the study's subjects. This sort of selective presentation—whether it was a product of the paper's reporting and editing process, or a consequence of the identity of the volunteers the study's authors decided to make available to the press—further slanted the content of the story toward its unwarranted conclusion.

An accurate summary of the results of the study would have read something like this: "Obese people who lose little or no weight can cut their risk for diabetes by more than half by engaging in moderate exercise and eating a healthier diet. Researchers studied three thousand people who had an average BMI of 34, which means they weighed 38% more than what the federal government currently considers a maximum healthy weight. Three years after entering the study, the average subject had lost only 8 pounds, and still had a BMI of 33, that is, a weight 33% higher than what the government recommends as a healthy maximum. Despite losing little or no weight, the subjects who exercised and changed their diets reduced their risk of acquiring diabetes by 58%—far more than the reduced risk acquired by subjects who took a drug designed to prevent the disease. The study provides yet more evidence for the view, held by a growing number of researchers, that improved fitness and a healthy diet, rather than weight loss, are the keys to good health for people at all weight levels."

I looked at numerous media reports regarding this study, and not one featured anything even remotely resembling the above summary. This should not have come as a shock. After reading dozens of stories about similar studies over the course of the past couple of years, I should by now be fairly inured to their pattern. And yet somehow, these stories still have the power to shock that part of me that clings to the belief that you can count on sources like the *Wall Street Journal* (and the *New York Times*, and *Harper's*, and so on) to present the undistorted facts on weight and health. Time and again, I find myself playing the role of an investigative Charlie Brown, racing up to kick the football Lucy is about to pull away. When, I wonder, will I finally learn that this is simply the way things are when it comes to reporting the facts regarding weight in America today?

The way things are almost requires that, when a large-scale study measures the effects of certain lifestyle changes on health, and those effects are discovered to be profound, the reporting of this information will focus instead on statistically trivial levels of weight loss. Time and again, the pattern of these stories does not change: Formerly sedentary people become physically active, start eating healthier diets, lose little or no weight, and enjoy drastic improvements in their health. Somehow, the moral of these stories almost always becomes some variation on "losing just 10 pounds can cut the risk of developing X in half."

Again, this study, like so many similar studies, provides no real evidence that weight loss *by itself* has any beneficial effects. After all, the volunteers lost so little weight, on average, that a significant proportion must have lost no weight at all, or must have actually gained weight. The bottom line is that most of the study's subjects did almost nothing that actually managed to alter their weight, which remained substantially unchanged. They were solidly "obese" when they began the study, and they remained that way. Only in a culture positively obsessed with weight could anyone imagine that altering one's BMI from 34 to 33 would, in and of itself, have significant health effects of any kind. Think of it another way: How plausible is it that *gaining* 8 pounds over the course of three years would, by itself, *increase* a person's risk of contracting diabetes by nearly 60 percent?

Consider that the volunteers in this study lost an average of 3 ounces per month, which is the caloric equivalent of eating one less saltine cracker per day. They did, however, do a great deal to alter their sedentary lifestyle and poor dietary habits. And the overall health benefits they enjoyed from *these* changes were immense. Yet somehow, according to the *Wall Street Journal*, these facts add up to the conclusion that "weight loss is the best defense" in the battle against Type 2 diabetes.

That is the message that all but a few readers of one of our nation's best and most widely read newspapers most likely took away when they encountered this major story summarizing the latest research regarding a disease that affects roughly fifteen million Americans, and that some predict will strike perhaps twice as many over the course of the next few decades. It is a message that certainly serves the interests of the nation's fifty-billion-dollar-per-year weight loss industry. It is a message that gives America's compulsively thin upper classes yet another reason to look down on the fat maintenance workers who sweep up copies of the *Wall Street Journal* left on the seats of our nation's commuter trains and jetliners. And it is a message that plays a crucial role in propping up the central justification for our rapidly intensifying war on fat—that fat kills.

In the end, there is only one problem with this message: It isn't true.

9

The Endless Debut

IN HIS STUDY of Spanish life in the 1960s, James Michener relates that one evening he was sitting with a friend, a middle-aged Spanish man, on a bench in the plaza of a Spanish town. The two men were watching the *paseo*—the informal ritual in which couples walk around a town's plaza in the cool of the evening. Michener's friend commented on what he described as "the beautiful sight of all these fat Spanish women." Michener asked him what he meant. "In America," his friend explained, "you have divorce. So American women need to stay thin. In Spain, there is no divorce. So after Spanish women get married, they get fat. Of course their husbands often acquire mistresses, but they would do so in any case. At least our women can eat what they want." That was nearly forty years ago; and although in the years since Spain has become, in regard to both divorce and weight, somewhat more like the United States, the story still captures an important truth about America's self-defeating war on fat.

Michener's anecdote alludes to a crucial factor that helps explain the fear and loathing fat elicits in America today. The culture of divorce plays a key role in fueling the war on fat, for a simple reason: In a divorce culture, even people who have been married for many years are always just a step away from being back on the marriage market. This fact creates a pervasive social climate that might be called "the endless debut." By contrast, in more traditional cultures young people go through a relatively short period of time between adolescence and adulthood, during which it is expected that their physical desirability should be at its peak. In such cultures it is understood that youth does not last. Generally speaking, after spending a few years courting and pairing off, adults in these cultures are not expected to maintain particularly youthful appearances.

Modern society has reversed that expectation. In this regard, contemporary America bears more than a passing resemblance to Huxley's *Brave New World*, in which the upper classes employed every technological device available to maintain the appearance of youth all the way up to the point of death. In our own brave new world, upper-class Americans spend untold hours in the "health" club, and billions of dollars on cosmetics and surgery, to produce a weak simulacrum of the same effect.

The extent to which Americans have become obsessed with maintaining a youthful appearance is most evident in the films we produce. Consider four well-known actors, and their respective appearances in the following films: Sean Connery as James Bond in *Diamonds Are Forever* (1970); Pierce Brosnan as Bond in *The World is Not Enough* (1999); Anne Bancroft as Mrs. Robinson in *The Graduate* (1967); and Sigourney Weaver as Gwen DeMarco in *Galaxy Quest* (2000).

When he made *Diamonds Are Forever* Sean Connery had not yet turned forty. Yet by today's Hollywood standards, he plays a character who appears to be close to sixty: Balding, wrinkled, and paunchy, there is nothing even remotely youthful about Connery's appearance. Connery, of course, has always been considered something of a sex symbol; and thus it is particularly significant that thirty years ago, when he was the highest paid actor in the world, he felt no need to appear to be younger than he actually was. By contrast, the Bond of Pierce Brosnan, who was well into his mid-forties when he made *The World Is Not Enough*, appears to be about twenty years younger than Connery's 007 in *Diamonds Are Forever*. This shift reflects a general Hollywood trend. Actors such as Sylvester Stallone and Arnold Schwartzenegger have gone on playing action heroes until their fiftieth birthdays and beyond, by following strenuous workout and diet regimens that (along with cosmetic surgery and various tricks of the film trade) allow them to maintain the appearance of men many years younger than they actually are.

Among female actors, this trend is even more pronounced. Many people have noted how Hollywood films rarely feature leading roles for female characters much older than twenty-eight. Over the past two decades, many leading actresses have reacted to this situation by maintaining an eerily youthful appearance. In the mid-1960s, when Anne Bancroft played Mrs. Robinson, she was a thirty-six-year-old playing a character whose age, while not specified, must have been around forty-five. And indeed she looked forty-five—a dangerously sensual forty-five, but forty-five all the same. Compare that character to Sigourney Weaver's character in *Galaxy Quest*. Weaver, who was fifty when the film was made, is playing a character in her late thirties, and could easily pass for twenty-eight. Weaver is just one of many Hollywood's leading women who, by dint of endless hours of work with personal trainers and/or the regular employment of cosmetic surgery, have managed to maintain the faces and bodies of women in their twenties for decades.

Now it is true the film industry is a world unto itself—but it is a world that has an enormous influence on the rest of the culture. Americans spend tens of billions of dollars per year on products that promise to help us mimic the look of perpetual youthfulness that is crucial to the celebrity culture. This money is spent on cosmetics, surgery, exercise equipment, miracle diets, diet foods, diet books, diet videos, and, most of all, drugs of every kind: drugs whose makers assure us will restore our hair and our sexual potency, remove our wrinkles, give us the energy of youth, or keep us eternally slim. (The latest craze along these lines is represented by Botox parties, at which mildly drunk yuppies convince each other to use a drug that for around five hundred dollars will remove their wrinkles for a few months.) We are, in short, encouraged to live our lives in an endless debut, in which the pursuit of a youthful appearance remains at the center of our lives until close to our dying day.

Indeed the pragmatic reasons for this are fairly compelling. In a culture in which it has become more or less acceptable to dump one's mate in the pursuit of self-actualization, to fail to combat the outward signs of aging—especially gaining weight, which many people have a strong tendency to do from the age of about twenty-five until around sixty—is to court disaster. One unintended consequence of the universal triumph of no-fault divorce has been to force millions of Americans to ask themselves regularly, "If I were back on the market, what would my prospects be?"

American women have been asking themselves that question for a

long time. For all the changes wrought by feminism, a glance at contemporary popular culture reveals the extent of the anxiety that still
surrounds the question of acquiring and, even more important, "holding" a man. The recent film version of the best-selling novel *Bridget
Jones' Diary* captures that anxiety particularly well. Bridget Jones is
supposed to be a fully self-sufficient adult, with her own career and all
the traditionally male concerns and ambitions that go along with it.
But every one of her diary entries begins with a simple three-digit
number: her weight as of that morning. This is followed by a catalog
of her caloric intake from the previous day, along with comments regarding how "good" or "bad" she managed to be. The substance of the
entries reveals that she is obsessed by two topics: her inability to consistently maintain an "ideal"—deeply unrealistic—weight, and her inability to find a suitable man (in her mind these two topics are, for
practical purposes, one and the same).

In the film version the character of Bridget Jones is played by a
conventionally slim actress (Renée Zellweger), who made headlines by
being willing to gain weight in order to become "fat" enough to play
the role. In fact, Zellweger gained 20 pounds, so that she played the
role while weighing 129 pounds (she is about 5'4"). That, in a nutshell,
captures America's obsession with weight today: A 109-pound actress
of average height gains 20 pounds to play the role of a "fat" 129-pound
woman—that is, a woman who would not be considered fat in almost
any other culture, past or present—and is subsequently congratulated
for the bravery it must have taken to sacrifice so much for her art.

And while it remains the case that the effects of the endless debut
continue to fall disproportionately on women, it is also true that men
are becoming increasingly subject to many of the same pressures. For
obvious reasons advertisers and their clients would like to condition
men to become as neurotic about their appearance as women have
been taught to be. Recent statistics pointing to an exponential growth
in cosmetic surgery procedures for men seem to confirm that this goal
is beginning to be achieved.

A pair of recent television advertisements reflect what could be
characterized as the increasing objectification of the American male.
The first advertisement is for Propecia, a topical solution designed to
stop hair loss. Viewers see a thirty-ish man, who, reflecting the cultural ideal for men, is both slim and muscular. The actor may have the
slightest hint of a receding hairline, but this is probably an illusion

suggested by the context of the ad. In any case, he is shown in a montage of playful exuberance with his conventionally beautiful wife/girlfriend (model-thin; long, shimmering hair; about twenty-five years old). In the voice-over, we hear his character say: "Will she still feel the same way if I lose my hair? Sure she will . . ." [We then see her flash a suggestive look at some obscure object of desire—her man? A rival?]. "She'll just feel that way about somebody else!" Although the tone is lighthearted, this message isn't intended as a joke, as the remainder of the sales pitch makes clear. The message is quite straightforward: Do what you can to retain your looks, or prepare to lose your woman to another man.

An even more striking example is provided by a recent Diet Coke advertisement. We see a thirtysomething man pushing a grocery cart through a supermarket, accompanied by his small children. They are clearly having a lot of fun together. The voice-over is provided by his wife: "He may not have time these days to spend hours running, or at the gym, chasing some image of a guy with a thirty-two-inch waist [actually, the actor playing the husband appears to have about a thirty-three-inch waist]. But he has time for more important things [at this juncture, we see him put a six-pack of Diet Coke in the grocery cart]. What he doesn't know is that the guy he is now blows that other guy out of the water."

Again, the message could hardly be delivered with less subtlety: It's OK if you, the domesticated husband, no longer have a perfect body because of the burdens of domestication. After all, you can still maintain a *nearly* perfect body—by drinking Diet Coke.

This sort of thing is becoming so culturally pervasive that even texts whose overt message rebels against precisely this type of objectification often end up reinforcing it. Consider the scene in the film *Fight Club*, in which the characters played by Edward Norton and Brad Pitt board a city bus, the upper inside wall of which features what looks like a typical Calvin Klein male underwear ad. Norton's character's voice-over comments: "I began to feel sorry for men packing themselves into gyms, trying to look like Calvin Klein or Tommy Hilfiger said they should look." His character then nudges Brad Pitt, points to the ad, and says, "Is that what a man is supposed to look like?" Pitt's character laughs, and responds sarcastically, "Self-improvement as masturbation."

It is typical of the surreal world of contemporary Hollywood that

Brad Pitt, of all people—he of the legendary abdominal muscles—
should be making this comment. On its surface *Fight Club* is a protest
against the superficiality and narcissism of America's consumer culture; yet at the same time its almost overtly homoerotic celebration of
an extraordinarily stylized version of male physical beauty manages to
subvert that message quite effectively. In other words, it's OK to laugh
at America's obsession with appearance—if you happen to look like
Brad Pitt.

Advertisements and images such as these suggest that men are being encouraged to become obsessed with the need to maintain a
youthful appearance and the associated level of sexual desirability.
The message is now being driven home constantly in advertising, in
films, and on television: Don't lose your hair, don't get fat, and you
won't find yourself back on the market. Naturally, as a man, I consider
this trend appalling. There is, however, an argument for the proposition that it's a good thing. Perhaps after men have been subjected to a
sufficiently oppressive cult of narcissism, with its attendant emphasis
on the quest for eternal youth and an unattainable body, the chances
will improve for reversing the culture of the endless debut, with its
poisonous insistence that we should all strive to remain thin, toned,
and twenty-one for the rest of our days.

No one, after all, actually *wants* to remain on the market for the
rest of his or her life. Recognizing the fundamental fraudulence of the
war on fat would be an important step toward undermining the notion
that there is some sort of health-related justification for striving desperately to look even a little like Brad Pitt (who, remember, is technically "overweight") or Gwyneth Paltrow. For the narcissistic pursuit of
eternal youth has nothing to do with health—quite the contrary.

When he reached his eightieth birthday, the French writer Paul
Claudel commented: "Eighty years old! No eyes left, no hair, no teeth,
no legs, no wind! And when all is said and done, how astonishingly
well one does without them!" Compare that attitude with our own hysteria toward getting old in general, and toward getting fat in particular.
In the end, the culture of the endless debut will not save us from
growing old—but it can prevent us from growing up.

IO

Chronic Restrained Living

THE FRONT-PAGE STORY in the January 2, 2001, edition of *USA Today* has a headline just made for a feature published on the day after New Year's: "There Is a Way to Keep Off the Weight." What secret formula has been found, we are supposed to wonder, what magic elixir or recondite method has been discovered, that will allow America, as it pushes its groaning belly away from the holiday feast, to enter into that Holiest of Holies, the Temple of Perpetual Slenderness?

Answer: dieting. Of course it isn't called dieting. After all, we all know that dieting doesn't work. The name for the newest cure to what ails us is "chronic restrained eating," or CRE. Predictably, the weight loss industry's latest marketing tool sports the sort of pseudoscientific acronym favored by the newest generation of diet gurus, as they peddle old ideas in new book covers to their increasingly plump and desperate readership.

CRE, the story informs us, is not a diet. It is, rather, "a general philosophy about food." This "philosophy" consists, essentially, of encouraging people to develop an obsessive-compulsive attitude toward food and eating. "People who practice CRE to manage their weight are constantly vigilant about what they eat: They often eat less than they want, plan their meals ahead of time, and think through what they'll eat before they go out to dinner, attend a party or sit down to a big family dinner," the story informs us.

If you think this sounds exactly like a diet, that's because it is. While CRE doesn't feature some of the more outrageous claims of the classic low-carbohydrate or low-fat or low-sugar diets—all of which contradict each other—the idea at the core of CRE is exactly the same as that endorsed by all diets: Eat less than you want to eat, and don't eat many of the things you would most like to eat at all. At bottom, CRE is a product of the fact that, in the wake of several generations of almost total failure, the diet industry has discovered "diet" is becoming a four-letter word—and so they are busily coming up with euphemisms for diets, diet books, diet foods, and so forth.

Thomas Wadden, director of the Weight and Eating Disorders Program at the University of Pennsylvania School of Medicine, explains why he believes in the virtues of CRE: "Most people have to be chronic restrained eaters to maintain a healthy weight," he informs the ever-credulous American public. "They have to eat less than they'd like to, and eat less than they are being urged to eat by neighbors, friends [and] advertisements."

Inquiring minds might want to know why it should be necessary to make the consumption of every bite of food a matter of hyper-vigilant concern, merely to maintain a "healthy" weight. Shouldn't a well-functioning body signal to its occupant when he or she has had enough to eat? Not necessarily, explains James Hill of the University of Colorado. Hill is a cofounder of the National Weight Control Registry, a group of three thousand people who answered the NWCR's plea to hear from people who claim have lost at least 30 pounds and kept it off for a year or more. "For most of mankind's history, we haven't had to regulate our body weight," says Hill. "It's something that happened naturally. But in the current environment, if you let it happen naturally, you become overweight or obese. If you trust your instincts, you'll overeat and under-exercise. You have to override your instincts."

Hill is actually a relative moderate in the diet wars, but these particular comments capture much of what is wrong with mainstream obesity studies. First of all, while it's true that for most of mankind's history human beings were rarely fat, it is also true they usually had a life expectancy less than half of that enjoyed by people in the United States today. This, of course, is not an argument for the proposition that being fat extends life (although, as we have seen, being 75 pounds "overweight" does not hurt life expectancy as much as being 5 pounds "underweight"). Yet obesity researchers rarely seem to be given pause by the fact that life expectancy and obesity rates in America have been rising in tandem for at least a century now.

Americans are constantly getting fatter and living longer, in part because of declines in smoking, which in addition to slicing years off their lives has always helped people stay thinner than they would otherwise be. Now it remains possible that fat is a significant health risk, and that the parallel increase in life expectancy and obesity rates is a product of factors that more than cancel out the health risks of fat. Nevertheless, at the very least the fact that the fat "epidemic" has yet to produce any visible effect on overall life expectancy—other than to correlate nicely with its increase—ought to create more skepticism about claims that fat kills than such assertions usually engender. Phony health scares always feature endless warnings that we are "about" to see the dire consequences of whatever. In regard to weight, the current apocalyptic predictions that America is eating itself to death are essentially identical to those issued by various public health authorities twenty, and thirty-five, and fifty years ago. Consider this passage from Roberta Seid's excellent history of America's obsession with weight, *Never Too Thin*:

> Medical spokesmen deluged the professional and lay press with their pronouncements [about the dangers of excess weight]. Dr. James Hundley of the National Institutes of Health declared that "high blood pressure, heart disease, diabetes and a shortened life span are all associated with obesity." The following November, in a *U.S. News & World Report* article entitled, "Danger of Being Too Fat," Dr. Hundley answered the question, "Is excess fat really dangerous?" with an emphatic, "There is no question about that. It is." "Obesity has replaced vitamin deficiency diseases as the #1 nutrition problem in the United States today," Dr. W. H. Sebrell, Jr., Director of the National Institutes of Health, announced. Dr. Lester Breslow, Consultant to the President's Commission on the Health Needs of the Nation, made a similar proclamation and stressed that even "normal Americans" are [now] so heavy "that [their weight] is inducing excessive mortality." He urged that all Americans strive for the weights deemed desirable by the Metropolitan Life Insurance Charts. The press informed the lay public about the

unsettling news in a barrage of articles, like the *New York Times* piece entitled, "Overweight: America's #1 Health Problem." For the rest of the decade, these dire warnings continued unabated. Scientists were unequivocal. Overweight shortened life. Dieting and weight reduction lengthened it. "Pleasingly plump" was not just unfashionable. It was deadly.

The "rest of the decade" meant the rest of the 1950s. Indeed, by 1960 nearly half of the adult population of the United States had become "overweight," according to the definition of that term employed by today's public health establishment. No trace of the public health calamity that was supposed to be an inevitable consequence of this epidemic of fatness has ever materialized. It is a tribute to the perennial character of America's obsession with weight, and the power this obsession has to suspend media skepticism, that the same dire predictions continue to be published, generation after generation, with no notice given to the fact that the predictions never show any sign of coming true.

Furthermore, our latest surge of panic over what by now must surely be the longest-running "epidemic" in medical history is largely a product of statistical manipulation. Because the population's weight follows a standard distribution—that is, a bell curve—placing the definitions for overweight and obesity near the populace's median weight guarantees that an average weight increase of just a few pounds will suddenly throw millions of Americans into the overweight and obese categories. This is precisely what happened during the 1990s, when an average weight gain of 8 pounds among American adults produced a 61% increase in the obesity rate.

The American experience merely parallels what is happening all over the world: Economic development invariably leads to less malnutrition, a more sedentary lifestyle, higher rates of obesity—and far longer life expectancy. Much attention has been given recently to the fact that Westernization has caused an "obesity epidemic" in the developing world. For example, there are islands in Micronesia where over 80% of the adult population is now obese. Prior to Westernization the life expectancy on these islands was less than forty years, in part because the threat of starvation was constant. In the past few decades, as Western foods and medicines have made their way to these islands, life expectancy has improved dramatically. One consequence of this is that these people are now living long enough to die of heart disease—a development that predictably enough anti-fat researchers attribute to the "obesity epidemic" that wasn't plaguing these islanders when their average life expectancy was thirty years lower than it is today. In other words, affluence causes both obesity and far better overall health. This in turn suggests strongly that, whatever negative health effects may be attributable to obesity, they are trivial in comparison to the health benefits conferred by the economic changes that make populations heavier.

Obesity researcher Paul Ernsberger points out that a similar story has occurred among the Pima Indians. "The Arizona Pima," he notes, "are the fattest people in the world, with an average BMI over 30, and very high rates of diabetes." By contrast, the Pima of northern Mexico, who are genetically indistinguishable from those in Arizona, live on the verge of starvation and are therefore much leaner and seldom suffer from diabetes. Their life expectancy is also much less than that of their Arizona cousins. "Should the benefits of Westernization be withheld to prevent obesity?" Ernsberger asks. "Or is it better to live fat than to die thin and malnourished?" Our anti-fat warriors would reply that it's better to enjoy the benefits of Westernization while remaining thin, conveniently overlooking the fact that, even if this as yet untested hypothesis were to prove true, no one has managed to devise a method of producing this result that actually works for any but a small minority of people who employ it.

The fact that until very recently almost all human beings lived in the shadow of starvation has certain consequences for those who wish to lose weight in societies where food has become cheap and abundant. Our bodies are well adapted to the threat of starvation: Deny the body food and it will go into a famine mode in which it expends fewer calories while waiting for food supplies to become plentiful again. And, when it is in this mode, it will send out increasingly strong signals that it wants fat and sugar—the substances best suited to helping the body get through a period of caloric scarcity.

For dieters, the consequences of these biological facts are well known. After an initial period of relatively easy weight loss, it becomes increasingly difficult for dieters to lose weight, and increasingly easier for them to give into intense cravings for high-calorie foods. Eventually, the vast majority of dieters give up. Many of these people find it almost impossible to return to normal eating patterns: Instead, they binge on foods rich in fat and sugar, which the body, as it comes out of famine mode, converts into fat to prepare for the next famine. This is the theoretical mechanism behind the empirical fact that dieters often end up weighing more than people who started out at a similar weight but never began dieting in the first place. And, as we have seen, yo-yo dieting is far worse for health than simply maintaining even very high levels of body fat.

"Someone needs to say that the emperor has no clothes," says Wayne Callaway, an endocrinologist and obesity researcher at George Washington University. "What we're dealing with here is cultural bias, not science. Obesity researchers have been ignoring everything we know about biology, which is that people adapt, and since for most of human history we've adapted to starvation, it's natural that some people are heavier now. Instead, we've been doing this weird ironic experiment: taking affluent people and making them starve."

Also, contrary to Hill's warnings, it's safe to say that the one thing Americans never do when it comes to food is "trust their instincts." Living in a culture in which they are bombarded by radically contradictory messages about food and body image—in which they are implored to "supersize" their fast-food meal and to fit into a size zero—few adult Americans (especially women) have enjoyed anything like "natural" instincts regarding food in a very long time.

Hill believes that a small number of Americans don't have to worry about their weight, because they are genetically protected from gaining "too much." He also believes that an even smaller number of Americans will be fat no matter what they do. One does not have to be a strict social determinist to ask the following question: If, as Hill and other orthodox obesity researchers believe, nearly two out of every three adult Americans weigh too much, while living in a culture in which weighing "too much" brings with it severe social condemnation, poverty, job discrimination, poor self-image, and a host of other well-documented disadvantages, why would anyone believe that a significant proportion of those people could actually manage to acquire and maintain more socially acceptable bodies? Do these researchers actually believe American culture is too *tolerant* toward fat? What basis, in other words, do obesity researchers have for believing Americans could be substantially thinner than they in fact are? After all, for most heavier-than-average Americans weight loss that was both significant and permanent would require staying on some sort of diet for the rest of their lives—and if medical science has established anything about weight loss, it is that very few people can manage this.

In this regard CRE is less disingenuous than most traditional diets, in that it openly admits requiring its adherents to sign up for a lifetime sentence. As diets go, CRE's message is unusually straightforward: If you can manage to eat less than you want to eat, and little or none of many of the foods you would most like to eat, almost every day for the rest of your life, you will lose weight and (probably) manage to keep it off. In other words, CRE is merely an acknowledgment of the grim truth that diets only work if you stay on them forever.

To which a nation of dieters (115 million Americans are dieting on an average day) might well be tempted to reply, thanks, but we already knew that.

Some people, of course, can actually do this. Not many—there is something about CRE that goes against almost every healthy instinct a human being has—but a few. The star of the USA Today story is a 5'11" sixty-one-year-old professor of civil engineering who limits his daily food intake to 2,100 calories, walks several miles per day, lifts weights, and does calisthenics—and still weighs 190 pounds (technically overweight, according to the ever-helpful government BMI tables). The engineering professor "jots down the calories of the foods he eats in his daily planner . . . [and] has learned how many calories he burns in a day by visiting a scientific laboratory that was able to help him figure it out . . . If he wants an ice cream cone, he (occasionally) has a small one . . . He eats only his favorite kinds and doesn't settle for less than the best." It goes without saying that the feasibility of maintaining this Spartan routine largely depends on having the sort of time and money available to academics and other professionals, but not to the fat working-class and poor people whose polyester stretch pants horrify the delicate sensibilities of the upper class.

Unsurprisingly, the professor claims he is subjecting himself to a lifetime of dieting bondage for health reasons. "I figure," he says, "that this is the key to longevity, health and vigor." As we have seen, the professor is wrong about that, but how is he to know, when so many obesity experts are assuring him that he needs to engage in this sort of behavior in order to maintain a "healthy" weight?

Yet as usual, the truth will out. The story concludes with the revelation that the professor "was heavy as a child and teen and knows the unpleasant social consequences of being overweight. That motivates him. 'Nothing works for the long term except restrained eating,' [he] says. 'I'm very disciplined. The fact is that not gaining weight and remaining healthy is more important to me than indulging.' "

This is what we have produced in America today: a society in which a sixty-one-year-old male engineering professor—that is, a person of considerable status and achievement, of the gender acculturated to invest a relatively small amount of its sense of self-worth in personal appearance—is still so haunted by emotional wounds inflicted in childhood and adolescence that he has spent a lifetime not eating what he wants to eat. Is it any surprise that he rationalizes the deep sadness that has driven him to live this kind of life by clinging to the notion that he has done all this in order to maintain a "healthy" weight?

When Jacqueline Onassis was dying of cancer, she complained bitterly to her friends about the sacrifices she had made to stay "fit" (is it possible to imagine Jackie O fat?). "Why did I do all those push-ups?" she wanted to know, when cancer was killing her at the age of sixty-four. Indeed, much of the health and fitness cult in America is driven by a subconscious belief that people who die have committed some basic error in their workout routine, and/or have eaten one too many Twinkies. Listen to a conversation among middle-aged professional persons, especially one full of fitness buffs or food fascists, about the death of anybody under eighty. The subtext of such conversations brings to mind the scene in Tolstoy's *The Death of Ivan Ilyich* in which the elegant Schwartz greets Peter Ivanovich at Ivan Ilyich's wake: "Schwartz was just coming downstairs, but on seeing Peter Ivanovich enter he stopped and winked at him, as if to say 'Ivan Ilyich has made a mess of things—not like you and me.' "

None of which is to deny that maintaining an active lifestyle is important. To the contrary, as Steven Blair points out, Americans have "a misdirected obsession with weight and weight loss. The focus is all wrong. It's fitness that is the key." And as we have seen, it simply isn't true that maintaining a "healthy" (sic) weight will improve either your health or longevity. Except at the statistical extremes, weight has little or nothing to do with basic health and fitness; on average, fat active people will be as healthy as thin active ones, and much healthier than thin sedentary individuals.

But suppose this were not the case. Suppose that the traditional view among obesity researchers is—despite the weight of the currently available evidence—eventually vindicated. Would it still be worth it to be a chronically restrained eater—a person who writes down everything that he or she eats, and adds up the calories at the end of the day? (Recall that even the crude statistics of large-scale epidemiological studies, which do not take into account such crucial variables as sedentary lifestyle, fail to show that most "overweight" and "obese" people have significantly higher mortality rates than thinner people.)

But let us take those crude statistics on their face. In general, they indicate that a person who would be considered quite "obese" in America today—say, a 5'4" white woman who weighs 215 pounds— would have a life expectancy of perhaps two years less than a woman who is 5'4" and 150 pounds. (It's important to note that this latter weight, although it is probably just about the statistical ideal, would still be considered "overweight" by most American women, and by the health agencies of the federal government.) Also, we shouldn't lose sight of the fact that the 215-pound woman will still have about the same life expectancy as a 5'4" 110-pound woman, and a better life expectancy than a 100-pound woman of this height (again, all of this is being estimated at the crudest level of statistical analysis). The 215-pound woman will have a much better life expectancy and health prognosis than any of these other women, if she is moderately active and they are sedentary.

Nevertheless, let us assume that the simplistic world inhabited by orthodox obesity researchers correlates with reality, and fat does indeed "kill" with the level of efficiency reflected by these statistics. Is the prospect of a year or two of extra life worth several decades of daily denial? Is spending hours every day in what CRE enthusiasts describe as a state of "constant vigilance," planning and calculating the caloric damage of every meal well ahead of time, agonizing about whether today is the day that one can allow a morsel of brownie to pass one's lips, or whether one will be able to resist temptation at the salacious wedding buffet, "worth it"? Worth what, exactly? Remember, that extra year or two of life, should you be so lucky as to enjoy it, is not an extra year of childhood, or youth, or middle age. Somerset Maugham claims somewhere that the pleasures of old age are not inferior to those of youth—only different. That always sounded comfortably plausible to me. As I enter my increasingly creaky forties, however, I'm beginning to have doubts about this particular dictum.

But let us also assume that Maugham is right—that a year of declining old age is in its own way as precious as a year of golden youth. Are fifty or sixty years of slavery to the false gods of slenderness (although not of *real* slenderness—fashionably thin people die sooner than all but the very fattest among us) worth the reward that may come from spending ten or twenty thousand days in bondage to the food diary and the calorie counter?

The question almost answers itself. No, in the end CRE—which, at the most fundamental of all psychological levels, means chronic restrained *living*—is not really about health or longevity at all. It is about being called "fatso" on the playground. It is about not having a date for the prom. It is about seeing an idiot in an Italian suit or a size 4 dress get a promotion, while your own work goes unnoticed.

Everyone, at some level, understands this. The constant blather about how being thin is a matter of "health" and "fitness," whether it emanates from the government agencies, or the obesity researchers, or the diet scam artists, or for that matter from your own mother, is all an elaborate facade that fools nobody, but stays firmly in place, because in regard to these matters the truth is something that is simply too painful to face.

Frederick Exley's memoir *A Fan's Notes* is a passionate and often beautiful polemic against everything associated with chronic restrained living. A novelistic re-creation of what he describes as "that long malaise, my life" it ends with a lyric, almost mystical vision, as he contemplates, from the perspective of the late 1960s, the future of America's golden youth:

> Like cinema starlets who have only recently been manufactured, they are precisely like one another: all six feet two; all have fine, golden complexions; all have that admired short hair molded formally to their pates; and all are dressed in button-down shirts topped by V-necked cashmere sweaters, below which they sport iridescent Bermudas displaying youthful, well-made legs. Looking at them, I see they are the generation to whom President Johnson has promised his Great Society; the generation which will never know the debilitating shame of poverty, the anguish of defeat, the fateful irony of the unexpected disease; the gen-

eration that will visit the barren moon and find it, because they have been conditioned to find it, more lovely than that river which, though so close to it, they cannot even see; the generation which will all retire to the great American Southwest, where under dry, brilliant, and perpetual suns they will all live to be a hundred and fifty, watching reruns of Ed Sullivan on a colored screen twenty feet high. What I am now certain I am beseeching them to consider is that of itself longevity is utterly without redeeming qualities, that one has to live the contributive, the passionate, life and that this can as well be done in twenty-six (hence Keats) as in a hundred and twenty-six years, done in no longer than the time it takes a man to determine whether the answer is *yea* or *nay*.

Exley drank himself to death by his mid-sixties (when told he had only six months to live, he reportedly replied "Great! Six more months to drink!"). And of course the excess and dissipation of the narrator of *A Fan's Notes* should not be taken as a model for healthy living. Yet one need not be a drinker with a writing problem to still hope that there will be more days than not when the contributive, passionate part of one's soul would trade a year or two of old age in return for the gifts necessary to have written something as eloquent as that.

On the other hand, the fate of Keats, who was tubercular and therefore fashionably thin, might be a harder pill for even the most fame-crazed writer to swallow.

> This living hand, now warm and capable
> Of earnest grasping, would, if it were cold
> And in the icy silence of the tomb,
> So haunt thy days and chill thy dreaming nights
> That thou would wish thine own heart dry of blood
> So in my own veins red life might stream again,
> And thou be conscience-calmed—see here it is—
> I hold it towards you.

Would I trade fifty years of life in exchange for having written that, or "Ode to Autumn," or "La Belle Dame Sans Merci?" I doubt it. Nevertheless, despite my partial enslavement—which, dear reader, is in all likelihood not so different than your own—to the insane cult of thinness masquerading as "health" that besets our nation, I think (or hope?) I can say with the confidence the affirmation deserves that I would much rather pay such a price for such a reward, than forgo a lifetime of passion in return for nothing more inspiring than a few more miserable months of chronically restrained life.

II

The Athlete Within

I'M WATCHING a package of highlights from the 2000 National Football League season. Many of the highlights feature the winner of the league's Most Valuable Player award, St. Louis Rams' running back Marshall Faulk. The NFL's MVP from this season scored twenty-six touchdowns, in part because he is one of the league's fastest players. Time after time, Faulk is shown accelerating away from speedy defensive backs, using his almost world-class sprinter speed to make a shambles of the schemes designed to stop him, or at least slow him down.

According to the U.S. federal government, Marshall Faulk is obese. Mind you, he is not merely "overweight"—every single running back in the NFL is "overweight." At 5'10" tall and 211 pounds, Faulk, along with one hundred thirty-one of the league's other one hundred eighty running backs, has a body mass index of more than 30. More than half of the league's players are "obese," including not only all of the offensive and defensive linemen, but more than three-quarters of the linebackers and tight ends, as well as the brilliant young quarterback Daunte Culpepper, who, despite (or rather because of) his weight, is considered one of the two or three most dangerous runners among NFL signal callers.

With one exception, all of the league's other one hundred six quarterbacks are "overweight"—that is, they have a BMI of at least 25. In fact 97% of the players in the NFL are either overweight or obese. Even sixty-six of the league's seventy-five kickers—traditionally the position reserved for pencil-necked soccer players—are "overweight." How is this possible? How can it be the case that this large group of superbly conditioned athletes, who have reached the pinnacle of America's most popular and physically demanding team sport, can be so fat?

Several explanations suggest themselves, none of them complimentary to the traditional assumptions of obesity studies. As we have seen, the BMI tables themselves, despite the almost sacrosanct status they have been given within the war on fat, are largely useless for making meaningful predictions about the relationship between weight and health. Except at quite severe extremes, body mass by itself has no value as a health and mortality predictor once other variables (especially activity levels) are taken into account. Indeed, some proponents of the BMI tables have begun to admit this indirectly, when they caution that the tables are not as relevant to "athletes," because athletes tend to have relatively low percentages of body fat in relation to their overall weight.

The idea, you see, is that it isn't weight itself that is harmful: It's fat. As is so often the case in the peculiar world of obesity research, this bit of supposedly scientific wisdom turns out to be the precise opposite of the truth. Apparently many of the health problems thought to be associated with "excess" weight are actually associated with large quantities of lean body mass. In their comprehensive review of the literature, Paul Ernsberger and Paul Haskew describe this phenomenon:

> A variety of evidence indicates that excess lean body mass or muscle is more hazardous than excess fat. Hypertension has long been thought to be related to excess lean tissue as well as to excess adipose tissue. [Examinations of thousands of patients] found that most of the apparent effect of weight on blood pressure could be accounted for by increased blood pressure in broad-chested individuals, because increasing weight had little effect on blood pressure within each body-build group. Blood pressure increased with weight in the group with slight build, but blood pressure actually decreased with weight among those with the broadest build . . . Thus, excess lean body mass, not excess fat tissue, may be associated with in-

creases in blood pressure and cholesterol . . . Excess lean body
mass may contribute to other cardiovascular diseases . . . in addition, excess lean body mass has been linked to breast cancer.

The authors cite several studies indicating that, among heavy individuals, high percentages of body fat may, on the whole, be healthier
than high percentages of muscle. Intriguingly, they point to evidence
indicating that fat people may gain the same cardiovascular benefits
from relatively low levels of exercise that leaner athletes gain from
higher levels, because of the greater work involved in moving their
greater body mass: "Cardiovascular function in fat people resembles
that in athletes, who also exhibit increases in lean body mass, plasma
volume, and resting oxygen uptake."

Ernsberger and Haskew also quote a review of the literature on
cardiovascular disease, asserting that "all that is now known about the
response of the heart and circulation to work indicates" that the idea
that the excess weight fat people carry strains the cardiovascular system "is false for obesity and cardiovascular disease." Indeed, this review suggests that, rather than encouraging fat people to lose weight,
"there is more evidence for a proposal to add a weight pack to improve
cardiovascular function by increasing circulatory work."

The authors conclude from this and similar evidence that "the Pro-
crustian impulse toward a one-size-fits-all rubric for health flies in the
face of common experience. The natural range of human size and
shape extends far beyond the confines of the Metropolitan Life tables
of 'desirable weight.'" They also point out that the belief thin people
are thin and fat people are fat because of a simple relationship between the calories people take in and those they expend has no basis
in medical science: "Light-boned ectomorphs barely alter their weight
despite hearty appetites, while endomorphs and some mesomorphs
burgeon as they age despite normal caloric intake."

In lay terms, some people are born with bodies that will one day be
ideal for running sub-four-minute miles, while others have a genetic
makeup that predisposes them to develop into great football players.
The idea that Marshall Faulk and Sebastian Coe (the 5'11" 120-pound
former world-record miler—that is, an athlete who weighs 100 pounds
less than Faulk, proportionate to height) should, if they wish to be
healthy, strive to weigh within 10 pounds of the same "ideal" weight is
completely unsupported by any scientific evidence. Yet this is what the

federal government, at the behest of the obesity research establishment, advises Americans to do.

Of course very few people are born with the sort of athletic talent
that can be developed to world-class levels. But that does not mean
that the less athletically gifted cannot be athletes. An "athlete" isn't
just someone who can run eight hundred meters in 101 seconds or
score twenty-six touchdowns in an NFL season: From a public health
perspective, an athlete is anyone who is physically active enough to
garner the immense health benefits that come from being active. And,
as the work of Steven Blair and his colleagues at the Cooper Institute
indicates, that level of activity is actually quite modest.

One of the most discouraging statistics that emerges from America's
misguided war on fat is how few Americans engage in enough physical
activity to qualify for the Cooper Institute's "moderately active" category. People in this category, which the Institute's research indicates
comprises a level of exertion that provides most of the enormous
health benefits derived from avoiding a sedentary lifestyle, engage, in
the course of an average day, in physical activities that are at least
equivalent to a single, brisk half-hour walk. Qualifying for this category certainly doesn't require that one take part in formal exercise. Any
kind of moving around counts: walking the dog, taking the stairs, gar-
dening, mowing the lawn—basically anything that can get a person off
the couch and out of the car. Yet only around 30% of the population
qualifies for even this modest standard! (Only 10% qualifies for the
highest fitness category, equivalent to taking a brisk hour-long walk
perhaps five times per week.)

There are many reasons why Americans find themselves living in
one of the world's most sedentary cultures. An economy built around
desk jobs, a social structure based on driving, the proliferation of elec-
tronic amusements that have pushed aside traditional outdoor games
for so many children—all these factors and many more have played
their part. Yet perhaps the biggest single factor has been the perverse
focus of the war on fat, which remains obsessed with fatness rather
than fitness, even though, as we have seen, there is no necessary contradiction between these two conditions. Regular exercise is crucial to
health—along with not smoking and not being a substance abuser, it's
one of the three most important things anyone can do to maintain
good health—but, as millions of Americans have discovered, it's not a

particularly good way to lose weight (since there are no good ways to lose weight, this is hardly a criticism of exercise).

People take up aerobics, or running, or bike riding and, when these activities fail, as they usually do, to give them the body their culture has taught them to want, they become discouraged and quit. Worse yet, many larger-than-average people, especially women, give up regular physical activity because they have been told that the key to good health is to lose weight, and regular exercise does not produce this result for them. They feel intimidated by gyms full of women with relatively "ideal" bodies (of course most of these women are deeply dissatisfied with their bodies as well), so they are often discouraged from trying to exercise even before they begin.

Fortunately, fat activists such as Marilyn Wann have begun to spread the word that it is perfectly possible to be fat and fit. In her wonderfully polemical book *Fat!So?* Wann sums up the principles of the nascent fat fitness movement:

> If you want to live a long and healthy life, you don't need some fad-diet-guru-optimization-lifestyle book to tell you how . . . You already know the answer. It can be summed up in four words: Eat right and exercise . . . The hard part, the part you will probably resist with everything you've got, the part that could turn your world upside down (in a good way) is the part where you stop hoping to lose weight. That hope has nothing to do with health or with living a long and happy life and even less to do with real hopefulness. Wishing your weight would change is about conformity and self-hatred and insecurity and prejudice, and everything that's designed to bring you down.

Those words, if they could somehow be read and understood and accepted by everybody in America who believes they need to lose 10 or 30 or 75 pounds, would do infinitely more good than any "cure" for fatness being cooked up in the labs of orthodox obesity researchers and the pharmaceutical companies that support them.

Countercultural rebels such as Wann, as well as distinguished scientists such as Steve Blair, Paul Ernsberger, and Glenn Gaesser, have already discovered the cure for the disease of obesity. The cure for this disease is simply to recognize that it doesn't exist. There is nothing wrong with Marilyn Wann, just as there is nothing wrong with Marshall Faulk, or any other "obese" person (or thin person for that matter: according to the federal government Sebastian Coe ought to try to gain at least 15 pounds) who is physically active, eats a nutritious diet, and is in good general health. None of these people has a weight problem. The people with the weight problem are those who construct and worship elaborate monuments to pseudoscience such as the BMI tables, based as they are on the absurd idea that there is such a thing as an "ideal" human weight, for all people everywhere.

In the summer of 2001, I took part in a one-mile road race in downtown Boulder. After participating in the men's "Masters" division, I stood at the edge of the course near the finish line to watch the men's open division. Soon, a pack of superb runners blew by me, led by a Kenyan who is one of the world's top marathoners. Yet not long after, I saw an even more amazing sight.

He was fat. Not heavy-boned, not well-muscled—but rather flat-out fat, with a huge gut and thighs that were easily twice as big around as mine (and I don't have a classic runner's body, by any means). He was about my height—5'8"—and he must have weighed at least 240 pounds. There were runners of the same height in this race who weighed literally half what he did. Yet he was ahead of most of them. He looked as if he might be what in Mexico is known as a *mestizo*—a person of mixed Spanish and Indian ancestry. His long jet-black hair was tied into a ponytail that was flying in the wind behind him.

As he approached, I couldn't believe how fast he was going. He looked like a runaway locomotive, or some NFL linebacker's nightmare of a giant fullback, bearing down on the defense with a full head of steam. I glanced at the race clock: He was going to cross the finish line a full minute faster than I had, with a time better than that of 95% of the runners who had participated that evening in the various waves of this race.

A passage from *Ulysses* ran through my head—a line about a thoroughbred, a long shot, winning the big race: "A dark horse flashes past the winningpost, his mane moonfoaming, his eyeballs stars." Suddenly I found myself shouting for this runner, shouting for him as the crowds shouted for Sebastian Coe on that summer evening in Oslo when he shattered the mile world record, urging the great athlete on, as he sped through the Scandinavian twilight into athletic history.

12

Why Do Americans Diet?

OF ALL THE MYTHS that surround the issue of fat in America, the one that has reached the most Orwellian proportions is the idea that Americans are (and should be) committed to losing weight because they are concerned about their health. This is an example of an assertion that continues to be treated as true precisely because it is so false that any acknowledgment of the depth of its mendacity would be even more disturbing than the falseness of the assertion itself. It is, in other words, a perfect example of the power of the Big Lie to survive scrutiny, when far less egregious falsehoods cannot.

Consider the facts this claim ignores or denies:

1. There is at present little or no credible medical evidence that, for all but a small percentage of Americans, increased weight represents a significant independent health risk.

For the vast majority of larger-than-average Americans, there is very little evidence that weight represents any sort of significant independent health risk. Being heavier than average *may* be a sign of the presence of other factors that *are* health risks, especially a lack of physical activity, but there is no real evidence that weight itself causes undue health problems, at least not until one reaches a level of body mass that is more than 100 pounds above the average for persons of a particular height. Indeed, even among people who have been labeled "morbidly" obese by the medical profession (this term is usually used to refer to persons who weigh more than twice as much as the "ideal" [sic] weight for their height), it's often difficult to find evidence for the proposition that their weight is a significant independent variable in regard to their health. Only when people reach weights that begin to render them nearly immobile does the case for the proposition that fat is an independent health risk become well documented.

2. There is at present no credible medical evidence that losing weight is a desirable strategy for maintaining or achieving good health.

As Glenn Gaesser has put it, "of all our convictions about health, 'thinner is healthier' has no rival when it comes to the gap between belief and evidence." Even if it were true that fat could be shown to be a significant independent health risk for more than a very small percentage of the population, it would not follow that attempting to get fat people to lose weight would be a sound medical strategy. Only the crudest sort of pseudoscientific reasoning would conclude that, because condition X is associated with people who have trait Y, eliminating trait Y in those people would necessarily eliminate condition X. For example, light-skinned persons are many times more likely to develop melanoma than dark-skinned individuals. On the basis of the reasoning that drives the case against fat, light-skinned people should all get deep suntans, in order to acquire the lower risk of melanoma enjoyed by darker-skinned people (in fact, for lighter-skinned individuals in particular, prolonged exposure to the sun greatly increases the risk of contracting melanoma). It is simply not known whether heavier people who become and remain thin thereby acquire the health risks of people who were thin in the first place.

3. Even if it were shown that "excess" weight is a significant independent health risk, and that losing weight would lessen that risk, it would make sense to try to lose weight only if the benefits of attempting to do so outweighed the costs.

In fact, it has become clear that the health benefits, if any, of losing weight do not outweigh the health costs of attempting to do so.

Note that, as a matter of public health policy, it makes no sense to separate the theoretical question of whether it's desirable for people to lose weight from the practical question of what actually happens when they attempt to do so. Yet in the war on fat it is routine for public health officials to treat these as if they were wholly separate issues.

As we have seen, the reason it isn't known whether people who lose weight and keep it off acquire the health risks of people who have always been thin is that, in order to test this hypothesis, it would be necessary to run a series of clinical trials that have never been run successfully. In these trials, a statistically significant group of fat people would lose weight, and keep it off, while another group would not lose weight. Researchers would then compare the long-term health of the first group to that of the second.

The reason no such trials have been run is that there is no known method to get a statistically significant group of people to lose weight and keep it off. Of course a small minority of individuals manage this feat, but the vast majority of people who attempt—even under direct medical supervision—to lose weight eventually gain all the weight back; indeed, a large percentage of these people end up weighing more than they did prior to their weight loss attempts. And the evidence has become compelling that this process of attempting to lose weight and failing to do so is far more damaging to health than maintaining even very high weight levels. In short, while the health risks, if any, of fat per se remain largely unknown, the health risks of attempting to lose weight are both clear and significant. If Americans were aware of the relative health risks of being fat and of dieting, and if they were actually trying to lose weight in order to improve their health, no one would ever go on a diet.

But *do* Americans try to lose weight primarily in an attempt to improve their health? There is a great deal of evidence that health concerns play an insignificant role in America's fifty-billion-dollar-per-year weight loss industry. For instance, diet drug combinations such as fen-phen, which have killed some of their users, are pushed through the regulatory process with relative ease, while millions of Americans eagerly swallow both the pills and the accompanying propaganda of the diet industry that fat kills—not because there is any reason to believe fat is more dangerous than fen-phen (quite the contrary), but rather because much of the public is willing to run serious health risks in the pursuit of cosmetic weight loss.

Diet books all pay lip service to the scientifically unsupported idea that their readers should lose weight to improve their health, but predictably enough they show no interest in the considerable body of research indicating that the benefits of an active lifestyle and healthy eating habits are largely independent of weight loss. This omission has become especially striking, given the diet industry's recent effort to repackage itself in terms of selling "lifestyle changes" rather than "diets." (In the cartoon series *Pinky & the Brain,* the title characters try to move the Earth, only to discover it's too heavy. Brain: "How are we going to get the Earth to lose weight?" Pinky: "I know! We can get everyone to go on a diet!" Brain: "Diets don't work." Pinky: "Not even if you call them 'A Whole New Way of Eating'?" Brain: "No.")

Still, the diet industry could never get away with its distortions if the industry's customers were interested primarily in health, rather than in cosmetic weight loss. Under such cultural conditions, the combination of the industry's failure rate and the absence of evidence for the claim that weight loss is beneficial to health would destroy the market for weight loss products. Similarly, without an enormously profitable market for cosmetic weight loss, obesity researchers—who in theory are committed to doing research designed to improve peoples' health—would have long ago admitted that their field's orientation toward questions of weight and health was fundamentally misguided. (To their great credit, a growing number of obesity researchers have come to this conclusion, although one would never discover this by relying on the mass media's coverage of the issue. Naturally such researchers are, in effect, cutting themselves off from funding by the weight loss industry—and thus, as an institutional matter, "obesity research" itself rolls along largely unchanged.)

Perhaps the best evidence that people trying to lose weight are not motivated primarily by health concerns is provided by the profile of the typical customer of America's diet industry: a 5'4" woman in her thirties or forties who weighs between 150 and 170 pounds. As we have seen, there is no credible evidence that such a woman would improve her health by attempting to lose weight, or indeed even by successfully doing so. A typical set of statistics from a large-scale epidemiological study (the 1.8 million-subject Norway Study) illustrates this point. Those persons in this study who had a BMI of 26 to 28—which happens to be the average BMI of the typical American dieter—had the *highest* survival rate of any cohort. Indeed, while 70% of these people—all of whom would be defined as "overweight" by the U.S. government—survived to at least age seventy-five, less than 50% of the thinnest people in the study (those with a BMI under 18; almost all fashion models, for example, would fall into this category) survived to that age. Indeed, the thinnest people had essentially identical mortality statistics as the fattest people in the study—people who weighed, on average, more than 400 pounds!

The statistics from this study are typical of such surveys. The average American dieter, in other words, is in all likelihood *already* in the healthiest weight cohort—assuming, for the purposes of argument, that weight in and of itself has a reliably predictable relationship to health. When one then considers that losing and then regaining weight has been proven to be hazardous to peoples' health, it is difficult to avoid the conclusion that any doctor who would prescribe a diet regimen to a person with a BMI of 27 (i.e., to the average American dieter) ought to be considered guilty of what lawyers call per se (that is, automatic) malpractice.

An analogy can help clarify this point. In recent years, a number of studies have indicated that people who are light to moderate drinkers—who consume one or two alcoholic beverages per day—enjoy better health than people who don't drink at all. However, people who become addicted to alcohol suffer from far worse health than those who never drink; and indeed the health gap between alcoholics and abstainers is far larger than that between abstainers and moderate drinkers. Now imagine a culture in which the vast majority of people who drink at all become alcoholics. Surely everyone would agree that, in such a culture, it would be both irrational and extraordinarily reckless for the medical and public health establishment to encourage non-drinkers to drink alcohol, on the theory that people are better off drinking, as long as they don't become alcoholics. This is essentially the situation in America today in regard to the medical and public health establishments' attitude toward weight loss. (Actually the situation is even more irrational than this, given that, unlike in the case of moderate drinking versus abstention, there is no good evidence that heavier people will in fact enjoy improved health if they lose significant amounts of weight and keep it off.)

In order to gather more evidence regarding the extent to which the weight loss efforts of Americans are actually driven by health concerns, I conducted a survey of 273 people who are either currently attempting to lose weight, or have made concerted efforts to do so in the past. The group surveyed was overwhelmingly female (94%), predominantly white (88%, among the two-thirds of the respondents who specified their ethnicity), and had an average age of just over thirty-four years.

The respondents answered the following questions: (A) "If you could take a pill that would guarantee you would achieve, and/or continue to maintain, whatever weight you consider most desirable, would you take such a pill if it lowered your life expectancy? If the answer is 'yes,' how much life expectancy would you be willing to forgo?" (B) "If you could take a pill that would increase your life expectancy by five years, would you do so if such a pill also guaranteed that you would become (or remain) overweight? If the answer is 'yes,' how overweight would you be willing to become?" ("Overweight" was defined as any weight in excess of the respondent's ideal weight, however she or he defined this.)

The responses were revealing. In answer to the first question, 78% of the respondents said they would take such a pill. The mean number of years of life expectancy that those who answered yes were willing to forgo was 5.7, with a low of one year and a high of fifteen years. Even more remarkably, 91% of the respondents who answered question (B) in a useable fashion (210 of 231) said they would not take a pill that would increase their life expectancy by five years, if such a pill guaranteed they would become or remain overweight. Among the twenty-one who said they would take such a pill, the mean amount of weight they would be willing to gain in return for the increased life expectancy was 12 pounds, with a low of 5 pounds and a high of 25 pounds.

Some of the respondents included comments with their responses to the questions. Many of these comments tended to be along the lines of the following one, from a thirty-one-year-old woman I will call Kate: "I've never paid much attention to arguments about whether being fat is bad for your health. All I know is that being at the weight I've been at for most of the last five years [Kate described herself as '30 to 35 pounds overweight'] is bad for my emotional health. I just can't feel good about myself when I'm fat, even though part of me [knows that] being fat may not be in my control. I would gladly take such a pill, if it could make me thin."

In the abstract, it's easy to condemn Kate as a "shallow" or "weight-obsessed" individual. Yet if large majorities of American women respond to such questions in a similar fashion, this would seem to indicate that the problem is not individual but rather cultural. A few years ago, *Esquire* magazine conducted a survey that it claimed proved more than half of all American women would rather be hit by a truck than be 100 pounds overweight. It becomes easier to understand that preference when considering such data as that provided by a recent university study, whose authors placed two fictitious personal ads. One of the ads was supposedly written by a woman who described herself as "50 pounds overweight," while the other was purportedly written by a woman who described herself as a drug addict. The drug addict received 79% of the responses.

Why, we might wonder, do the related propositions that losing weight is good for one's health, and that most people who try to lose weight do so to improve their health, continue to dominate the public discussion of weight issues in America, when the evidence for both propositions is slender or nonexistent? I believe that, at bottom, the myths that fuel the war on fat survive in the face of the evidence because there are some truths that are simply too painful to face. How many of the 115 million people in America today who are on some sort of diet would be willing to admit that they have suffered, and continue to suffer, in the pursuit of a bankrupt (and largely unattainable) cultural ideal?

How much more comforting it is to tell ourselves that we are suffering in the pursuit of perhaps the most sacred of secular pursuits: the quest for health and longevity. In a culture in which it is the unstated premise of so much public policy that the main point of life is to stay alive for as long as possible, nothing could sanctify the war on fat more successfully than the widespread belief that attempting to lose weight is good for one's health. Actually, one thing would serve the purposes of that war even better: if this belief happened to be true.

13

The Last 10 Pounds

IN THE SPRING OF 2001, Denise Austin, one of America's better-known fitness gurus, published a diet and exercise book entitled *Lose Those Last Ten Pounds: The 28-Day Foolproof Plan to a Healthy Body*. As has now become the style in the weight loss industry, the author emphasizes that she hasn't produced a diet book, but rather a guide to making appropriate fitness and lifestyle changes. Apparently a century of consistent failure has finally produced enough public skepticism to require the repackaging of diets as something else—usually a "fitness" plan of some sort. Bill Phillip's bestseller *Body for Life* seems to have perfected the new formula, with its promise that the reader will have a "new"—that is, a much thinner and more muscular—body in just twelve weeks. (The highlight of Phillip's text is a series of implausible "before" and "after" photographs, which imply that any flabby middle-aged man or woman can be transformed into a potential fitness pageant contestant in less than three months.)

In comparison to some of its competitors, Austin's book is actually not all that bad. It tries to put as much emphasis on exercise as it does on dieting, and it even mentions in passing (a rare concession within the genre) that exercise has health benefits independent of weight loss. But make no mistake: The emphasis is still very much on losing weight, and the book's 1,500-calorie-per-day meal recommendations clearly constitute a very low-calorie diet for any adult who engages in the sort of "fat-burning" exercises Austin advocates. This level of caloric intake would create, conservatively speaking, a 1,500-calorie-per-day deficit for the average reader who followed the book's recommendations, which indeed is the level of caloric deficit necessary to lose 8—not 10—pounds in the advertised twenty-eight days. (Many nutritionists would consider a 1,500-calorie-per-day deficit a starvation diet.)

Of course the whole idea that the loss of "the last 10 pounds" has anything to do with what Austin's title calls "a healthy body" is ridiculous. In America today, dieters who are looking to lose anything like 10 pounds are almost invariably attempting to conform to a cultural ideal that is inimical to having a healthy body. A woman who weighs 10 pounds more than the current cultural ideal in all likelihood already weighs 10 or 20 or 30 pounds less than she would if she ate normally and exercised moderately. For such a woman, an ideally healthy weight would be precisely that: the weight she would maintain more or less naturally, by avoiding a neurotic attitude toward food, while engaging in moderate levels of physical activity.

In this regard, books such as Austin's are almost always disingenuous. Austin states that it isn't necessarily a good idea to make it one's goal to look just like the average woman one sees on television—like Denise Austin, in other words—but then she recommends a diet and exercise program that advertises itself as a means to achieve just this result. Austin's web page makes it even clearer than her book does that looking anything like Denise Austin would be, for the vast majority of women, something that would require a massive investment of time, effort, and money. (The web page gives examples of Austin's daily schedule, which includes somewhere in the neighborhood of two hours of vigorous exercise—roughly three to four times the amount necessary to maintain optimal metabolic and cardiovascular health.)

Indeed, the very concept of "those last 10 pounds," which is an extremely common one among dieters, reflects the deeply neurotic nature of America's obsession with weight and weight loss. Austin and her ilk claim to be promoting good health, but what they are really promoting is a mindset that is practically indistinguishable from that found among people suffering from eating disorders, especially anorexia nervosa. Consider the classic symptoms of anorexia, and then compare them to the mental state of many of the people (almost all women) who make up the bulk of the market for a book that promises to help its readers lose those last 10 pounds. (The numbered sentences are taken from a standard diagnostic description of the symptoms of anorexia nervosa.)

Anorexic individuals refuse to maintain normal body weight for age and height.

Again, most women who are attempting to reach or maintain a body weight that reflects the cultural ideal are already below—and often far below—their healthiest weight, that is, the weight they would maintain if they avoided regular bouts of semi-starvation behavior, and/or unhealthily compulsive exercise. In fact, a diagnosis of anorexia usually takes place only when such behavior becomes so extreme that it brings on an immediate medical crisis.

Although a few women can maintain a supposedly "optimal" BMI of 18.5 (for a 5'4" woman, this would be 108 pounds) without resorting to such unhealthy behavior, the vast majority cannot. Given the cultural ideals regarding weight that American women are currently expected to emulate, *Lose Those Last 10 Pounds* might be more accurately entitled *How to Engage in Anorexic Behavior without Becoming So Weak as to Require Immediate Hospitalization.* As we have seen, a woman who maintains a BMI of 18.5 when this is well below her normal body weight is a good candidate to suffer serious long-term health problems.

Anorexic individuals deny the dangers of low weight.

On the basis of this classic symptom of the syndrome, much of the American health-care establishment, not to mention all of the weight loss industry, could be said to be in the grip of a fundamentally anorexic state of mind. Despite a mass of epidemiological evidence that, in the words of one of the world's most eminent obesity experts, Ancel Keys, "underweight is a greater hazard than overweight," the average American concerned about the potential hazards of different levels of body mass will encounter hundreds of warnings about the potential dangers of fat for every such warning he or she encounters regarding the potential dangers of thinness.

How many Americans are aware that many large-scale studies on the effects of weight on health have indicated that a fashionably thin woman in America today has approximately the same long-term health prospects as a woman who weighs 300 or more pounds? Those who rely on the medical establishment for advice and information are unlikely to encounter such facts. For example, the famed Mayo Clinic has recently published a book entitled *Mayo Clinic on Healthy Weight*. This particular book isn't completely useless—it does warn its readers of the dangers of the most egregious fad diets—but it's packed with the usual alarmist misinformation about the supposed dangers of "excess" weight. Worse yet, the authors exploit the renown of their institution while informing readers that losing weight requires eating less and exercising more, forever, while at the same time ignoring the fact that almost all people who follow this advice in an attempt to lose weight and keep it off will fail.

The most interesting feature of this book is that, of its total of 208 pages dedicated to exploring the issue of "healthy weight," it devotes exactly one half of one of them to discussing the dangers of being too thin. The discussion of this topic is relegated to a shaded sidebar captioned "Are You Too Thin?" in which the authors go on to inform their anorexic readers (this is not a rhetorical description: who but an anorexic is going to be both too thin and reading this book?) that "you may be genetically thin," and that "it could be difficult for you to gain weight without gaining mostly fat. This would not improve your health." Yet the book's other 207 1/2 pages avoid any discussion of the fact that many people are genetically fat, and that it is going to be nearly impossible for such people to lose weight without gaining it all back (and more), which would not improve their health, either.

It's bad enough when so-called fitness experts spread serious misinformation about the benefits and risks of weight loss and weight gain. But when an institution such as the Mayo Clinic contributes to the construction and maintenance of an essentially anorexic attitude toward weight, the consequences are potentially much more severe. Lay readers depend on such prestigious institutions for objective medical advice; and, given the all-encompassing hold of the diet culture, few of them will ever realize they are being fed a diet of propaganda that is in many ways identical to that served up by the weight loss industry.

Anorexic individuals are terrified of becoming fat and of gaining weight; they report feeling fat even when they are very thin.

The struggle to lose those last 10 pounds is essentially a reflection of what is referred to in the eating disorders literature as "anorexic ideation," that is, the sort of distorted thinking that leads women who are already well below the average weight of women in almost all other cultures and times to see themselves as fat, or on the verge of becoming fat, or at least in serious danger of becoming fat if they do not maintain the "constant vigilance" regarding food recommended by the proponents of chronic restrained eating.

When someone such as Britney Spears is quoted as saying that there are mornings when she looks in the mirror and thinks "my butt looks fat," and that she has had to learn to "deal" with her bodily imperfections, and further, when such a quote resonates with the life experience of tens of millions of American women (and some men), it merely emphasizes the extent to which the mindset of an eating-disordered person has simply become the normal orientation toward food and body image for a significant percentage of women in America today. Significant pluralities, or in some cases actual majorities, of American women—especially, but not only, white upper- and middle-class women—freely admit to being terrified of becoming or remaining fat, and of feeling "fat" even when they are, by historical and cross-cultural standards, extremely thin.

Over the course of the last century, what has been considered the ideal body weight for American women has, making allowances for occasional fluctuations of fashion, been drifting constantly downward. The Gibson girl was thinner than the voluptuous ideal of the 1890s, while the flapper was thinner than the Gibson girl, and so on and on, reflecting a long-term trend that has produced the current age of Calista Flockhart and Kate Moss. (By way of comparison, although today we remember flapper fashion as being focused on boyish thinness—and indeed within the context of its time it was—the most famous flapper model was 5'7" and 140 pounds: almost zaftig by today's emaciated standards.)

Apparently the only practical limit to this ongoing process is that we have now reached a point where the cultural ideal for women's bodies is barely distinguishable from the bodies of women diagnosed with full-blown anorexia nervosa. On one level, the only difference between, say, the women actors on a television program such as *Friends* and the average anorexic, is that most women simply cannot be as thin as Jennifer Aniston or Courtney Cox Arquette without endangering their health to the point where they risk being hospitalized for an eating disorder. It is telling that, early on in that particular program's run, Aniston was reportedly threatened with the loss of her role if she didn't shed a number of pounds from her already thin frame. Subsequently other women actors have reported feeling "fat" whenever they see an episode of the program. An even more disturbing phenomenon manifested itself on *Ally McBeal*, in which Calista Flockhart starred. When the show became a hit, the other women actors on the program—almost all of who were already thin to begin with—began to lose noticeable amounts of weight. One of them admitted that she did so because she felt "huge" whenever she was on-screen with the show's star.

Anorexic individuals often engage in compulsive rituals, strange eating habits, and the division of food into good/safe and bad/dangerous categories.

Another term for this sort of behavior, of course, is "dieting." Anyone familiar with what Naomi Wolf has characterized as "the cult of dieting," and who has managed to escape that cult's grip will recognize that dieting, when carried out for any length of time, tends to devolve into a ritualistic and indeed obsessive-compulsive attitude toward food. As Wolf points out in her book *The Beauty Myth*, "women's magazines report that 60 percent of American women have serious trouble eating. The majority of middle-class women in the United States, it appears, suffer a version of anorexia or bulimia; but if anorexia is defined as a compulsive fear of and fixation upon food, perhaps most Western women can be called mental anorexics."

Evidence for the extent of mental anorexia—for the prevalence of something resembling the classic anorexic mindset that is vastly more common than the diagnosed incidents of the syndrome itself—can be found everywhere one looks in American culture today. Here are some examples from an Internet forum, a forum that is supposed to be devoted to discussions of the sport of running but that regularly veers off into arguments about food and weight loss (in fact most of the site's members seem to have begun running in order to lose weight).

One typical thread begins with the question, "How many sweets is too many?" The author of the original post (a twenty-three-year-old woman who describes herself as engaging in five to six hours a week of vigorous exercise) confesses that she cannot manage to cut sweets out of her diet completely, and then adds that she plans to start limiting herself to "one chocolate bar per week, and no treats at all in between." She wants feedback from the forum on whether this is reasonable, and on what sorts of limits others set for themselves.

The first respondent informs the poster that "a whole chocolate bar is a lot," and advises her to buy a bag of chocolate miniatures "and take two or three pieces to work with you. Don't take the whole bag." After reading this response, I half expect the respondent will be chastised for an obviously unhealthy attitude toward food, but far from it. The next respondent replies, "I agree . . . a whole chocolate bar is a LOT. Miniatures work very well!" This is too much for me, and I post a protest, pointing out how bizarre it is to criticize an extremely active young woman for choosing to eat one chocolate bar per week. I then advise the original poster to "stay away from people with eating disorders." (In doing so I assume this level of bluntness—not to say rudeness—will spare her from further advice along the lines she had been getting.)

Again, my naiveté in these matters is revealed by the next post, which deserves to be quoted in full: "Since you like at least one (1) candy bar a week, I'd cut it up into a bunch of little pieces so I can have a small piece every day. That's what I'd do. This way, you can have a taste without too much guilt, plus the pounds won't pile on. I like sweets but fortunately a tiny bit a few times a week at the most is enough for me." This post triggered an extensive argument among several forum members over whether an indulgence in one candy bar per week, for a young woman already burning an extra 4,000 calories per week through strenuous exercise, was or was not "too much"—as if this were a question that deserved to be debated rationally.

This debate took place within hours after someone describing herself as a 5'7" female distance runner posted a request for information on what a good running weight might be. When a respondent asked her what her body frame was like, the original poster replied that she didn't know, but that her dietician had prescribed a minimum weight of "106 to 107 in the A.M., which I hit today and I feel like a whale." (Estimates of the percentage of American collegiate female distance runners with eating disorders run to 80% and higher.) Fortunately this particular post drew a response from another distance runner who had suffered from anorexia nervosa, and who gave the poster some sensitive guidance on the topic.

Yet such is the depth of the neurosis surrounding issues of weight and body image in our culture that even this chilling glimpse into the surreal world of anorexia did not stop the forum's participants from almost immediately launching into a discussion of whether one candy bar per week was a permissible "treat" for a long-distance runner. Similar discussions seem to occur on this site (which in other respects is an excellent resource for information of interest to runners, thus making such discussions all the more uncanny) several times per week. Indeed, a forum participant responded recently to a sardonic suggestion that one of the site's forums be renamed "The Eating Disorders Training Clinic" by agreeing this wouldn't be a bad idea:

> I can't even *go* into [that forum] anymore because I simply *cannot stand* the encouragement of eating disorder behavior! Now granted, not everyone there is like that but I get so #&@$ sick of the same questions over and over: "I eat nothing but a carrot stick and a banana every day, run twenty miles a week, lift, bike, etc. . . . why can't I lose any weight?" Gee, I freaking *wonder* why not! "Why do my clothes fit more loosely but the scale says I gained five pounds? Isn't that bad?" "Do you think 600 calories is enough for me to eat and still lose weight?" Arghhh . . . I *had* an eating disorder for years, I *know* how sick that behavior is and destructive it is to your body!

The day before, someone had begun a thread actually entitled "Losing those last ten pounds," in which the poster asked whether it was possible to do so without being hungry much of the time. She was told that it wasn't, but was then reassured that "you will adjust" to a feeling of constant hunger. (This reply inspired the suggestion to rename the forum that in turn led to the response quoted above.)

In the end, the saddest irony of books like *Lose Those Last 10 Pounds* and forums such as this one (there are hundreds of others like it on the Internet) is that the logic of eating-disordered thinking precludes the possibility that there can ever be a last 10 pounds. This logic promises that when the weight-obsessed individual finally achieves a certain weight, she will be satisfied with the appearance of her body. But this is a false promise. An eating-disordered culture functions by making people deeply dissatisfied with their appearance, no matter what that appearance happens to be.

In Greek mythology, Sisyphus was condemned to roll a boulder to the top of a hill, only to see it tumble immediately to the bottom, over and over again, for eternity. The struggle to lose the last 10 pounds is a Sisyphean struggle, which is to say that it is an absurd task, in the existential sense of that word. America's dieters are, like Kafka's hunger artist, who longs for others to "admire his fasting," condemned to live in a world in which they are doomed to dedicate their lives to a task that can never succeed, and yet can never be abandoned:

> People grew familiar with the strange idea that they could be expected, in times like these, to take an interest in a hunger artist, and with this familiarity the verdict went out against him. He might fast as much as he could, and he did so; but nothing could save him now, people passed him by. Just try to explain to anyone the art of fasting! Anyone who has no feeling for it cannot be made to understand it . . . No one counted the days, no one, not even the artist himself, knew what records he was already breaking, and his heart grew heavy. And when a leisurely passer-by stopped and mocked the figure on the board and spoke of the obvious fraud, that was nothing but the stupidest of all lies, born of an indifferent and malicious heart, since it was not the hunger artist who was cheating; he was working honestly, but the world was cheating him of his reward.

14

Life During Wartime

I N THE COURSE of writing this book I interviewed more than four hundred people about aspects of their relationship to food, fat, dieting, body image, and our culture's obsession with these topics. The scope of the interviews ranged from fairly limited question-and-answer e-mail exchanges, to in-person conversations that lasted several hours. I have talked to, among others, very fat people, very thin people, thin people who think they are fat, people who would be considered thin in most other cultures but are labeled "overweight" in this one, people who are always trying to lose 10 pounds, people who have lost and gained back hundreds of pounds, people who have lost weight and kept it off, and people who have given up trying to lose weight at all.

I learned something from all these exchanges; many were fascinating. The interviews themselves highlighted how every person's story in regard to these issues is in some sense unique; but at the same time almost all these stories shared common threads. This chapter features excerpts from interviews of several people who have struggled with weight issues. I believe their voices are representative in that they reflect many of the major themes touched on in the stories hundreds of other individuals shared with me; but of course no selection or summary of such narratives can even begin to capture the full range of what it means to be fat, or think one is fat, or to fear being fat, in America today.

Perhaps the most valid generalization one can make about fat in America is that people who believe their own feelings about the subject are in some way unusual or extraordinary are almost always mistaken. I came away from many of these interviews with a sometimes overwhelming sense of the passion, the pain, and the anger this topic can elicit. Indeed I sometimes felt that, for many people, this was the single most important issue in their lives; and that, further, the issue had become nearly all-consuming in part because of a general taboo against admitting how important it can be. What follows, then, are a few voices from the front lines of the war on fat.

Rachel

34 years old, female; 5'3", 113 pounds. Law professor at a West Coast university.

"I remember the first time I experienced something like the adult emotion of depression. I was quite young, maybe nine or so, and my mother and I were going clothes shopping. I just kept seeing this chunky girl in the mirror. It made me reluctant to buy anything at all. I remember going home and lying on my bed and never wanting to shop again (I still hate shopping today—although for healthier reasons). I don't know exactly where my sense of the 'right' body type was coming from at that age. Probably everywhere. But during the summers my family went to a small beachside town where all the girls were skinny, blonde, freckle-nosed WASPs. My whole look was off—curly reddish hair, no freckles, olive skin. I was never fat, or even chunky, looking back on it. But I did not have those coltish, knobby-kneed legs either. It's sad to think that innocence about such matters ends when we are still such little children.

"Between nine and fifteen these feelings came and went, but I suppose they were gradually solidifying. I was a tomboy and athletically inclined, which helped a great deal. Also, I had a solid group of girlfriends until about the ninth grade, when a number of them switched to different schools. Then I had a summer job from hell that launched me into a decade-long pattern of eating-disordered behavior.

Would it have happened anyway? It's entirely possible. As I said, my problems with self-esteem with regard to looks had begun much earlier. And I should add that my mother, whom I love dearly and do not blame for what happened to me, was pretty nuts about being thin, as were most women of her age and social class. The epidemiology of these things is mysterious, however. The cultural factors are the overwhelming cause, but it probably takes just the right combination of circumstances to send an otherwise healthy, well-loved girl over the edge. That was me.

"Anyway, I was a mother's helper to a family that had hired me so that they did not have to spend the summer playing with their kids. We were living in their summer house, located in a beach town that was well below Newport or the Hamptons in terms of class status, but several notches above, say, weekends at Jones Beach. I was basically a house servant. The mother was an obsessive clean freak, so whatever time I didn't spend with her children I spent cleaning the house. The simple and short way to explain what happened is that I had no control over my life in any other way, so I started to exert enormous control over my weight. I remember being proud of the fact that the mother would marvel at how she could leave brownies out on the counter all day and I would never eat a crumb. I started to engage in all the classic anorexic behaviors—keeping a log of everything I ate; exercising to burn off anything I deemed as excess; refusing to eat any candy, sugar, or sweets of any kind, etc. Also, there was a group of mother's helpers who bonded during those miserable summer weeks, and one of our activities one day included bingeing and then drinking syrup of ipecac to make us vomit. Horrible things to learn. In retrospect, even the late-night drinking, bong hits, and Quaalude ingestions were better for us than that. By the end of the summer I weighed about 95 pounds. Lots of people worried that I looked too thin, but lots of people also complimented me. The fix was in.

"Of course no one can maintain the control that an anorexic does. Some can better than others, and they end up hospitalized or dead. For a combination of reasons, my behavior never approached full-blown anorexia nervosa. Again, athletics saved me to a large extent. I was a good athlete and needed energy to be on all the various varsity teams that I was involved with. In particular, I was a very good high school, and later collegiate, runner. While there is certainly a lot of running-inspired eating-disordered behavior, for me running was almost always a source of health. It forced me to eat enough to have muscles to run. It disciplined me not to binge and then purge when I was in competition. On the negative side, there is a terrible amount of body-image hysteria in women's distance running, complicated by the fact that it does help competitively to be very light, up to a certain point.

"At any rate, since I couldn't maintain the anorectic's control, my behavior slipped into an erratic kind of bulimia. For months, I would be relatively healthy in my eating—still always mindful to stay very thin, but not losing weight and not bingeing and purging. Then I would have very bad months. Daily binges and purges. Self-esteem in the toilet (pun intended). Shame and guilt about the very fact that I engaged in this disgusting behavior piling onto the self-loathing that caused it in the first place. Because I would have 'good' months, I would trick myself into thinking I was cured. Then when I was in a bad patch, I would say to myself daily, 'this is the last time, I am never doing this again.' How many thousands of times did I say that?

"It took me years, and the help of a therapist (whom I only saw for one crucial year in my early twenties), to stop the bulimic behavior. It took me even longer than that to arrive at a place where I truly have no issues with food. I credit my therapist, and also many women who have written many important books making the connection between sexism and women's body-image problems. Those books helped me a great deal. They depersonalized the issue for me in so many important ways. For so long, I thought I was just a freak who had no excuse for being so fucked up. For me, putting the issue in a political and cultural context was enormously important. Finally, getting more involved in various forms of physical activity in the outdoors helped too. Nature is a great antidote to culturally inspired neurosis. Who cares what you look like or what you ate, as long as you can make it up that next mountain pass?

"My biggest regret in life, and I try not to have regrets as a general rule, is that I lost so much time, so much energy, having this corrosive, destructive disease. I look back on pictures of when I was young now, and think, gee, what a cute kid. I never saw that then. And not seeing that somehow stopped me from doing so many other things in life that are wholly unrelated to how one looks. It's crazy. But that's where we live, isn't it? I am very fortunate in that I have many people in my life—my parents, siblings, friends, and now husband and children—who love me and think, and have always thought, that I am beautiful. I cannot imagine arriving at the place I am today without that support. I am also lucky in a much more shallow way. Today, although I never diet or count calories or avoid ice-cream cones, I am thin by conventional standards. I run and engage in other sports regularly, which helps. But a lot of it is dumb genetic luck. My family is, by nature, relatively thin and wiry. So it was in some sense easy for me to have reached this happy accommodation with my looks and society's norms. Yet the fact that this is so, and that for so long I was slowly destroying myself, says something powerful about how screwed up this culture is about weight. My one big hope in this regard is that my beautiful, funny, smart, fabulous daughters never have to go through what I, and so many other women, did and still do."

Joyce

34 years old, female; 5'7"; describes her current weight as "107.3 pounds," and adds unprompted both that her body fat percentage is 18%, and that this is "down 1% over the last four weeks."

"My current doctor tells me I need to gain weight, and I guess a part of me thinks that she's right, but I still can't bring myself to eat more. I'm forcing myself to eat 850 calories a day, and even that's a struggle. I like my body the way it is now. When I gain weight, I feel fat, and when I feel fat, I feel worthless. As a woman, my body is important to me. I've felt this way since I was fifteen. I'm happiest when I'm under 100 pounds, but I start fainting when I get below that weight for more than a few days, and my heart races a lot.

"When people ask me how I feel about food, I usually tell them that I try to avoid food altogether. I don't like food. I'm still trying to learn what a 'normal' weight is. This whole issue is very confusing to me. I'm trying to exercise, because I want to learn to see the extra weight I'm supposed to gain as muscle, not fat. I can't stand the idea of being fat. Even the word disgusts me. Overweight people want the world to accept them the way they are, so why can't people accept me the way I am?"

Sarah

26 years old, female; 5'2", 135 pounds.

"I'm always trying to lose weight. I know the acceptable thing to say is that I'm not interested in the number, and I try to tell myself I look fine. But I'm lying to myself.

"I have never been able to stick to diets, which I guess is OK, because I've always thought of myself as somebody who didn't fall for diet hype, especially the hype that surrounds the more faddish diets. I'm training for a marathon right now, so I'm doing a lot of research on how to eat right. But I would love to lose weight.

"Growing up, when my mother dieted the household dieted. Like I said, I couldn't stick to diets, but in high school I would sometimes starve myself for the entire day, or not eat anything until lunchtime. I also recently came across old diaries in which I congratulate myself for being good—eating frozen yogurt in a cone for lunch, that kind of thing. Because of my mother's involvement with Weight Watchers I have always looked at food in terms of exchanges—a fruit, a fat, a milk.

"I was always an athletic kid. In grade school, I always played sports. In college, I walked a lot, took several dance credits a semester, and ran off and on. Since then, I've taken up running much more seriously. In the last year I've completed three half marathons and a full marathon.

"When I first started running regularly I dropped a lot of weight (I got down to 118 pounds) and I felt great about myself. But right in the middle of my success I left the country to work for three months on a cruise ship. I ran a few miles every other day, but the general lack of activity in my day really took its toll. When I got back I had gained all the weight I had lost back, plus more, and my twenty-fifth birthday was approaching. I had a panic attack because I was once told that when you turn twenty-five it becomes so much harder to lose. And you know what? It has. Even after the three half marathons and the full, I can't lose the weight. I'm absolutely stumped.

"So I'm unhappy about my appearance right now. It's definitely important to me to maintain my body appearance—it's the only negative thing in my life right now. Thank goodness I've gained proportionately, so it's not really noticeable, but I'm unhappy. Pants that fell off my hips two years ago now barely fit. When I'm conscious of my weight or body image then I start to get depressed and it's harder to enjoy life. That could include everything from having a drink with friends to meeting a new client at work.

"I'm always comparing myself to others. I have kind of an unusual body: a 34D chest with a relatively small waist (26 inches), and larger hips (37). Up until I turned twenty-five I always had a completely flat stomach without ever having to work at it. I never did sit-ups. Marilyn Monroe was a perfect role model for me! I was really born in the wrong era.

"I think a big part of my self-consciousness about all this comes from my father. I recently came across an old diary entry where my father asked me how the food was at camp. When I told him it was lousy he said, 'Good, maybe you'll lose some weight.' I may not have been perfect, and I may have not made the best nutrition decisions, but I wasn't a *fat* kid. He made me feel like that, though. We no longer speak. . . .

"I have to say, though, that despite my recent (post-cruise) weight gain, running has changed my life. I shudder to think what would have happened to me if I had never started. At least now I'm working towards a fitness goal, and I can feel good about that."

Michael

41 years old, male; 6'3". Weight unknown: approximately 350 pounds.

"I wasted almost eighteen years of my life dieting. Most of my diets were self-designed, some based on engineering principles. I also tried various diets based on books and articles. I started dieting in high school, and kept the practice up until ten years after I was out of college. I wasn't constantly on a diet, but I spent the better part of eighteen years denying myself proper nutrition, and convincing myself that my life would be better, in one way or another, after I lost weight.

"Naturally I lost weight. Then I gained it back. Then I lost it again. This is the same pattern followed by millions of people. It is the pattern followed by those who have not yet realized that every weight loss attempt is doomed by the rules of biology—and the mathematics of homeostatic control systems—to ultimate failure. The weight will go away, easily at first, then gradually with more difficulty. But in the long run it is guaranteed to return. I refused to see this, and was destined to follow the same inevitable pattern.

"So, looking back on dieting, it was not only a waste of my time and energy, but it was doomed to failure. It lowered my self-esteem in inevitable and insidious ways, because the dieter is always taught to blame himself for the weight when it returns. Indeed, the main motivation usually employed to keep someone on a diet is to tell him or her how awful it is to be fat—to convince them that a fat person has less social value than a thin person. Dieters are taught to hate themselves in the guise of keeping them motivated to lose weight. And this guarantees that once a diet fails, the dieter will want to move on to the next sure-to-fail diet scheme.

"I had learned the lesson of self-loathing that every dieter is taught. I had convinced myself that my life would be better when I lost weight. At some point, however, I realized that I couldn't and wouldn't wait for a diet that would actually work. Instead I would accept my body's appearance, make reasonable changes to optimize what I had to work with, and make the most of my life. I decided that I had too many important things to deal with in my life, and I no longer wanted to waste precious time, thought, and resources on weight loss attempts. I realized I could achieve my other goals without first losing weight. Then, I realized that if I could achieve my other goals, there was no reason to lose weight.

"When I first had my epiphany, it was a lonely decision. Very few people I knew could appreciate or understand that I had decided that losing weight wasn't going to help me achieve my goals, and that it was really just getting in the way. It was another five years before I began to discover that there were other people—a lot of other people—who felt the same way I did.

"At first, the discovery of kindred spirits came through the Internet. I stumbled across a news group dedicated to people who were not trying to lose weight, but instead were trying to make the most of the life that they had while accepting and working with the body that was given to them. This was the first time I came across the formal idea of fat acceptance—the idea that you should accept yourself and your weight the way it is, and not wait for the diet to kick in before you made the most of your life.

"After I realized how much time and energy I was spending on weight loss attempts, I gradually began to see that the reasons normally offered as motivations to lose weight were hollow. The evidence that losing weight improved a person's health was flimsy. It was possible to attract women without being svelte—wit, confidence, sensitivity, and intelligence were far greater assets than physical appearance. And, as to physical appearance, it made a lot more sense to work with what I already had than to spend a huge amount of time and effort trying to make myself into something I might never become.

"For example, at one time, I exercised as part of my weight loss attempts. The real danger in doing that is that the weight will, inevitably, return. When it does, the victim decides the exercise 'isn't working,' that they are not achieving their goals, and abandons the exercise regimen. Now I exercise on a regular basis because it is essential to keeping my body healthy. It is extremely difficult for a fat person to exercise, because of the public ridicule that we are exposed to in most exercise venues. But I have learned to ignore that, and pursue a regular exercise program anyway.

"The worst discrimination I have experienced has been at the hands of the medical profession. I am forty-one years old, and I have lived in this body for over half the time that I am going to spend here. I am well aware of how it works, and what it is and is not capable of. I am well aware that it is not possible for this body to lose a significant amount of weight and keep it off for a very long time. I am also aware of the alleged health risks of being fat—and I have examined these with the trained critical eye of someone who makes his living in an engineering laboratory.

"Even though I know and have known for over a decade that the best thing for me to do is to leave my weight alone, and to allow my body to maintain a healthy, natural weight, I have yet to find a physician who will respect my decision—or who will treat me as anything other than a fat patient.

"I currently have no physician. I left the last doctor because he was subjecting me to a series of unwarranted tests, looking for ailments that fat people supposedly had. This is in spite of the fact that I had no indication of any of these conditions. He was obsessed with building a case for his 'syndrome.' The poorness of this science is astounding. First, assume all fat people have certain diseases. Then, test every fat patient for those diseases. But, don't test your thin patients. Then, when more fat patients are found with these diseases than (untested) thin patients, assume that the diseases must, somehow, be related to their fat. I couldn't respect a doctor whose analytical methods were so badly flawed.

"This isn't the first doctor I've 'fired.' I once had to quit seeing a doctor because of what happened when I went in to see her with a raging sinus infection. In spite of the fact that I was in agony, I received no medication for the infection, but got a lecture about my weight instead. I have to share a great line that I stole from someone on the news group. He said that if his wife went to the doctor with a gunshot wound, the doctor would tell her that if she lost weight she would make a smaller target. This, unfortunately, summarizes the attitude of most health professionals towards fat people and the subject of weight loss.

"It is almost impossible for a fat person to receive nonprejudicial medical care. I have no doubt whatsoever that this is the primary reason the health of fat people suffers. The second reason, of course, is that we are actively discouraged from exercising in public.

"I wish every fat person could be told about the National Association to Advance Fat Acceptance. This group has been around for more than thirty years, but I had missed their existence entirely. I only wish I had found NAAFA earlier. Now, I will tell everyone who will listen that there is an alternative to self-loathing and futile circular weight loss attempts. You can accept yourself, and you can accept the body that nature and its god intended you to have. Instead of working to change yourself in an unnatural way, you can work to change society to give you the rights and respect that you, and every other fat person, deserve."

Elaine

24 years old, female; 5'9". Describes weight as "fluctuating a bit between 135 and 142" pounds

"I am very, very muscular, and look much smaller than my weight (I wear a size 5).

"[In response to a question about her body fat percentage] I am not sure of my body fat, and I don't want to know because I know it will make me neurotic. Considering the margin of error, why freak out over something that has an accuracy of plus or minus 5%? Gosh, 5% is a huge difference! I do know that my body fat is low enough that I only menstruate about twice per year.

"I always wanted to lose weight, but I have really calmed down since I started running marathons. For some reason I would like to weigh in the 120s, but I am not sure why I picked that goal. I wonder what would happen if I achieved this—would I simply lower my goal?

"Growing up I was always an athlete, but for some reason I thought that I was fat. I was not. I remember being in elementary school and panicking when my family started shopping for a van. I was so afraid that somebody at school would say I was so fat that my family needed to buy a van to haul me around! What is crazy is that I was a popular, successful athlete and no one would ever say such a thing to me. It is helpful, I am sure, to understand that my very thin mother was once chubby and is anorexic and bulimic. She never binged, but she purged (laxatives) the very little that she ate.

"In our house we played the dieter's version of Trivial Pursuit—you start with all the pie pieces [in the board game Trivial Pursuit, each player has a six-piece miniature plastic pie mold that he or she fills up gradually with 'slices' by answering questions correctly] and instead of gaining pieces, you lose them. The winner was the one who lost the most. I also remember asking for a snack before going to bed and being told that it was good to feel hungry.

"None of the diets I attempted in high school (just general calorie-reduction diets—nothing drastic) worked until I came to college. I gained a lot of weight in my last year of high school and really did need to lose weight. The year of my crazy weight gain was the year my parents divorced and my mom was hospitalized for a month because of her eating disorder. I started running, and allowed myself less than 1,000 calories per day. I drank sugar-free Kool-Aid and coffee, and ate carrot sticks, air-popped popcorn, and sugar-free Jell-O.

"I hated that year of my life, and was thrilled to see myself slowly disappearing every time I looked in the mirror. I dropped about 80 pounds in six months. When I came home for the summer I was severely anemic and exhausted. I ended up gaining about 10 pounds, which I lost again over the next few years. My initial weight gain and eventual weight loss had more to do with my needing to feel in control of my life and general unhappiness than they had to do with my relationship to food.

"Anyway, for a number of reasons my body image is erratic and unstable. Some of these self-esteem issues have nothing to do with my weight, but have to do more with the fact that I grew up with an abusive father. If I am running well I usually feel pretty good about myself (control issue, I am sure). Sometimes I still feel fat—for no apparent reason, totally out of the blue. I don't talk about this much, but I do some sports modeling (no big deal—really), mostly leg stuff. I feel very weird about this and very few of my friends know that I do this work. When I first lost weight I hated how people (men, sexually, but women too, socially) suddenly changed how they treated me. Come on, guys! I am still the same person that I was then. Because of that, I don't like being evaluated based on my body.

"I don't really enjoy food—if I could take a pill that would give me everything that I needed to remain healthy I would gladly do that instead of eating. As I mentioned earlier, running marathons has really helped me calm down about my body. I usually run about sixty miles per week. I know that I will be lean as long as I am in training, and there is such a feeling of accomplishment from training for and running marathons that all of the encroaching feelings of doubt feel comparatively insignificant. I also know that if I exercise and continue to challenge myself both mentally and physically I will continue to feel more and more comfortable in my own skin.

"This is very important to me, because my preoccupation with weight has, in the past, interfered with friendships and my social life. I never want to go out to eat (why must everything revolve around food?), and at times I have felt too fat to fit in (which is ridiculous). I believe these self-esteem issues stem more from my violent relationship with my father than anything else—my body image, and my self-esteem issues surrounding it, is just how the emotional fallout from that relationship has manifested itself."

Julia

35 years old, female; 5'7", 167 pounds. Julia's background is in many ways strikingly similar to Susan Estrich's at the same age (see Chapter 16). She graduated at the top of her class from one of the nation's leading law schools, clerked for a Supreme Court justice, and worked for both a prestigious law firm and in an important federal government position, before becoming a law professor at an East Coast university.

"I've found that once I start thinking and talking about how bad this issue is—about things my mother has said to me, or what other people close to me have said—it becomes difficult for me to think about anything else. For example, a few months ago I was talking to

Alex [her fiancé at the time, whom she has since married] about Jason, a man I dated in college, and how I was thinner then than I am now, and Alex said something like 'oh lucky Jason.' We got into a huge fight over that, and we've spent hours since talking about the issue. Alex's previous girlfriend was both extremely thin and obsessed with remaining that way, and I needed him to understand that if that was his ideal, I was never going to be that. I've had endless discussions with him on this issue, looking for reassurance, which I know annoys him (it certainly annoys me—I'm not normally an insecure person).

"Discussing this reminds me of the time when I tried to share with my mother my feelings about how another man I had been serious about had become sexually uninterested in me, and her comment was, 'but you were fat then.' She said this in a way that made it clear she had no idea how painful that comment was: It was almost as if she expected this explanation and/or justification for his rejection of me to be so unexceptionable that I should just dismiss the topic from my mind.

"I struggle with the question of whether I should attempt to distance myself intellectually from this whole issue, or whether I should allow myself to get angry and impassioned about it. In some ways, it's like grappling with the relationship you had with your parents when you were a kid: Some people never seem to be able to get over the anger they feel towards their parents for things that were said and done years ago. They never leave home, emotionally speaking. But in other ways it's worse. After all, you can move away from your parents, at least physically, but you can't move away from your body. It's still here, every day.

"My father actually suggested I have liposuction when I was a junior in high school. I'm sure he didn't mean to be cruel or anything: My family comes from a background in which it's assumed that, if you have the resources to 'fix' some 'imperfection,' then you ought to fix it. No doubt he thought of liposuction for a fifteen-year-old girl as something like a nose job. And you know, the scary thing is, if I'm honest with myself, I have to admit that my parents really weren't all that bad in regard to this whole topic. They weren't *good*—but believe me, a lot of my friends have had it worse.

"My mother's side of the family is extremely thin. I strongly suspect my mother is anorexic: She goes for long periods without eating, and she talks about weight and weight-related topics constantly. Because of this, it's often very difficult for me to get through something as simple as a phone conversation with her.

"I think my parents' attitude had an effect on me in adolescence. I've noticed that most of my women friends today are around my size—around a 12. It wasn't like that in junior high and high school: I remember how in eighth grade my friends and I spent all summer drinking Diet Coke and doing 'thinner thighs in thirty days' programs—things like that. It was around this time that some of us tried to teach each other to throw up. Luckily, I think only one girl actually managed it—she's had a severe eating disorder in the years since.

"We were all thin, more or less, and looking back I realize now that we definitely excluded fat girls from our circle. You just weren't friends with 'fat' girls; I think on some level we were afraid it was contagious. More rationally, we all wanted to be popular, and being seen with fat girls wasn't cool. I wonder how many fat girls are fat because they're excluded, rather than the other way around?

"I know I was terrified of becoming fat. I basically lived by myself—my parents had jobs that kept them on the road much of the time—and so I would throw parties at my house all the time. I felt I had to do this to 'keep' my friends, because I didn't consider myself 'cute' enough to really belong to the popular crowd.

"Probably the most warped thing I can remember from that time was a summer camp in the mountains at which the counselors warned us not to drink river water, as you were likely to get Giardia. They explained this was a parasite that causes severe intestinal cramps and extremely painful gastric distress—you basically can't digest any food for days. Guess what? Within minutes half the girls were sneaking down to the river.

"Are you going to talk about clothes? Clothing designers are evil. What's fashionable today for girls and young women—low hip-hugging jeans and crop tops—is stuff that only Cameron Diaz can wear. Another thing you need to emphasize is the class angle in all this. There's a woman with whom I hung out in college, Jackie, who is very rich and wears size 4. She's had a nose job—all of her female relatives have had massive amounts of plastic surgery. One thing she has always loved to say about herself that just boggles my mind is that she has 'a great sense of style.' I tell her, 'Jackie, you're a size 4 and you wear five-hundred-dollar silk blouses on Saturday morning. Of course you have a great sense of style.'

"Then there's an old friend of mine who is constantly telling her stepmother that it's 'irresponsible' of her not to lose weight and have plastic surgery. Now, her stepmother is gorgeous: She looks fantastic for sixty-one, but my friend thinks she could look thirty-five if she set her mind (and her checking account) to the task. No doubt she's right about that, too. This friend has a two-year-old daughter, and the other day when I was visiting them the daughter sat down at the table, sighed, and said, 'I'm *so* fat.' Of course her mother (who is razor thin) says things like that all the time. It was hard to do, but I told my friend that if I heard her say things like that to her daughter in the future, I didn't think I could be her friend any longer. Maybe that will help—I don't know.

"I'm going to tell you something that is very difficult for me to discuss, as a woman who considers herself a strong feminist, and a supporter of women and women's issues. When I lived in San Francisco I went to a gay men's gym, and I loved it, because I wasn't judging the bodies of other women, while all the while knowing they were judging me in the same way. At the gym I go to here, if you tell me that there is a woman wearing a specific outfit on the stationary bike, I will know exactly whom you are talking about, without even looking. And I hate her. I hate the thin women at the gym.

"Worse yet, the other day I was watching a 'fat' woman—whatever that means—working out on a piece of equipment, and all I could think was, 'why is her butt jiggling like that?' The sight of her jiggling butt disgusted me—and then of course I immediately started thinking about the women who must feel the same way about me. And here we all are, stuck in this absurd hierarchy, hating the women thinner than us, and being disgusted by the women who are not as thin. It's such a powerful weapon for alienating women from each other.

"Here's another thing that's hard to talk about. Before I met Alex, the man I had been involved with was a guy who had just lost a lot of weight when I began to date him. He was an Atkins diet junkie, and an obsessive weight lifter. I stayed with him for four years—in fact I lived with him—even though he became emotionally abusive toward me. He never hit me, but he criticized me so constantly about my weight that my self-esteem was eventually all but wrecked. It reached a point where he refused to be in the same room with me while I ate. He said the sight of me eating was too much for him, and that we couldn't eat meals together until I lost weight.

"Only when he refused to eat with me anymore did I find the strength to leave him. Even so, I was a wreck for months afterwards. I couldn't catch a glimpse of my body in a mirror without feeling totally pathetic.

"The sad thing is that I had started to get healthier about these issues in the two years between college and law school. Now I wonder, is it just bad luck that I ended up with this creep, or did I seek him out because I have these issues? It's all quite complicated; still, it's been a real disappointment to me that some of my friends seem to minimize what he did, in a way they would never do if he had been physically abusive. Anyway, Alex seems really good about all this stuff. He understands now—does he ever!—how explosive the feelings that surround these issues can be.

"Here's how bad all this really is: You know how Susan Estrich said in that diet book that her proudest achievement was going from a size 12 to a size 6 dress? Even though she had been the first woman president of the *Harvard Law Review,* and the first woman to manage a major presidential campaign, and so on and so forth? Of course I think that was a terrible thing for her to have said in print. Yet I'm a size 12, too—and if I somehow managed to get down to a size 6, I know I would feel the same way."

Cynthia

52 years old, female; 5'10", approximately 375 pounds.

"That weight figure is a guess, because I haven't actually been on a scale in ten years or so. I was a fat baby, a fat kid, a fat teen, a fat adult, and now I'm nearing my dotage as a fat old bat. I no longer attempt to lose weight. At this point in my life I am unapologetically and unrepentantly fat. It's what I am—in the same way that I have red hair and green eyes. It's what I am—but not *who* I am. Being fat has certainly shaped the person I've become, but it's not the most important thing about me by any means.

"The funny thing is that when I finally stopped the diet/lose/gain/repeat-till-you-die cycle, I also stopped gaining. I have worn the same size clothes since shortly after my twins were born sixteen years ago.

This really was an eye-opener, because all the years I was dieting I believed that if I ever just stopped, I'd keep gaining until they had to cart my big butt around on a dolly. Nope. I gained to a certain point, and then stopped. Now this is both good news and bad news. The good news is that it seems my body, in its wisdom, knew where it wanted to settle in, and as soon as I stopped torturing it, that's just what it did. The bad news is that I have a strong suspicion this 'settling-in' point would have been a lot lower if I'd wised up a lot sooner.

"In the days when I did diet, I tried just about every one out there, at one time or another. Atkins, fasting, pills, Simmons, grapefruit, carb addicts, medically issued amphetamines and diuretics, lots of fruits and veggies, broiled meat, no meat, Lean Cuisine: I'm sure there are few, if any, that I didn't try over a thirty-year time span. Talk about self-abuse! I spent the majority of my life trapped inside that insane cycle. Someone should have had me committed. Isn't the definition of insanity doing the same thing over and over and expecting a different outcome?

"The first diet I remember was at about age ten. Physicians were giving me amphetamines and diuretics at twelve. Throughout high school, I dieted constantly and rigorously, but never managed to get below 200 or so pounds. I was active in sports—basketball, volleyball, all that—but I never managed to look like the other girls, and if I ever allowed myself to slack, it showed immediately in extra pounds. For me, exercise has always been driven by a desire to lose weight or just to prove I could. At this point in my life, getting from here to there is plenty of exercise. My knees are paying the price for those years of basketball and volleyball, and the same gene pool that contributed to my being fat has brought me some arthritic issues as well. Of my six children, three are thin, one is average, and two are heavier. All six have knee and other joint problems.

"As an adult, I continued the deadly, yo-yo cycle of diet, lose, and then gain back everything *plus* some. I'm sure that in my life I've lost and gained enough weight to make ten more people. The result of dieting most of my life was years of wasted energy, misery, and a sense of being an unmitigated failure, because no matter how hard I tried, and how much I brutalized myself, I could never accomplish what the 'establishment' said I would if I just showed some 'self-discipline.' Damn them all. They should have half the 'discipline' I imposed on myself in those years.

"It got to the point where I spent long periods of time on 500 to 700 calories per day or *less*. Eventually, there came a time when that was the only way I could lose weight. Of course, then there would be the 'plateau' periods where nothing—absolutely nothing—would cause one more stinking pound to disappear. By that time, my metabolism was so damaged from prolonged periods of starvation that I didn't need to eat much to gain weight. Keep in mind that throughout all this I never got below 230 to 250 pounds. I never did the binge-purge thing, but I did go through a period of using laxatives. In between diets I'd go back over 300. But desperate people do desperate things.

"At one point I joined Overeaters Anonymous, which as you may know is modeled on Alcoholics Anonymous. The problem was, I wasn't binge eating. Now I'm the first to admit that I eat things I could 'do without.' Who doesn't? No one really *needs* that chocolate dough-nut. But so what? A thin person wouldn't think twice about it. My thin children certainly don't. I just couldn't believe, and I still don't, that I was an out-of-control food addict. I was out of control, all right—but I was a diet junkie, not a food junkie.

"The problem with the alcoholic analogy used by OA is that an al-coholic can abstain totally from alcohol, but no one can abstain totally from food and live. Several times a day you need to sneak into the cave and pet the sleeping dragon. That's just the reality of it.

"About fifteen years ago, I finally came to the realization that I was on a futile quest. I was never going to fit the Madison Avenue stereo-type. So I made a conscious decision to stop it right then and there. Each one of us has only so much emotional and mental energy, and I decided that life was way too short to waste in such a shallow pursuit, and that my energy would be better invested in becoming more com-passionate, more loving, more generous, and in general becoming more in tune with the things I really value. I was no longer going to waste my life trying to meet some artificial standard that defined my worth as a human being by the size of my body. I would do everything I could to become a better person, and find ways to give something to my community—but not one more second would be squandered on trying to be thin: I might as well have been trying to fly to the top of the Chrysler Building.

"Enough is enough. I grew up a New York tenement kid: I stepped over winos and junkies every day on my way to school. That gives you an attitude that you don't lose entirely just because you move to a more scenic neighborhood.

"This isn't to say I still don't struggle with the messages society bombards us with: images of thin, air-brushed girls who have never even seen a stretch mark, much less had one. Those images tell us that this is what women must look like to be desirable. People like Jay Leno are utterly savage in gutting women like Monica Lewinsky in public for carrying a few more pounds than the 'average woman.' It isn't easy to stand in the face of the unrelenting humiliation that is heaped, without pity, on those of us who don't fit in the box.

"Over the years I have experienced the full spectrum of emotions regarding my size—from near-suicidal revulsion to acceptance. Do I still have days when I feel less than whole? Sure. Do I *like* being fat? No. Do I wish my joints didn't hurt so much? Yep. But I accept it in the same way someone who's 4'11" accepts not being 6'4", or that someone who has got alopecia accepts not having hair. But in general, it's not a problem for me any more. I deal with it as I would deal with any other physical characteristic that would require me to make accommodations. What is, *is*.

"My appearance is what it is. I can't control that. I am well groomed, well clothed, and that is as far as it goes. I'm well aware appearance matters because of the societal prejudice against fat people. The unspoken assumption is that fat people are undisciplined, lazy, smelly, and stupid. My college GPA was 3.94. I'm not taking a back seat to anyone, thank you. I was president of the Board of Education for three years, and I served on the Board of Directors of the state's Association of School Boards. I do not avoid the public eye.

"Certainly one of the major areas in which appearance is a factor is sexuality. Fat people are not asexual. When I stopped feeling sorry for myself I found that lots of men have a decided preference for big women. It's just a matter of finding them. They *are* out there. And anyway, fat is not nearly as unattractive as self-pity.

"Nevertheless, when one reads of studies in which very young children are shown pictures of other kids, including kids who are black or poor or in wheelchairs, and most of them say they would be least likely to want to be friends with the fat child—it's a knife in the heart. Where do they get these prejudices at such an early age? *Everywhere!* Their parents, at school, TV—simply everywhere, because fat is the last safe prejudice. We are urged to act compassionately towards people of other races, other cultures, and other abilities, but fat is assumed to be one's own fault and therefore a character flaw: something one should be ashamed of and ridiculed for. It's a damned lie.

"Let me tell you a story—just one of many. One summer, when my twins were about three, they were in a little wading pool in my front yard, and I was sitting on my porch steps watching them and enjoying the beautiful day. I was wearing jeans and a T-shirt. A white pickup truck with several guys in it drove by. The truck circled the block, and on the second pass it slowed and the man in the passenger seat hurled a bottle at me, shouting, 'Go back inside where you belong, you fat fucking bitch!' The bottle shattered on the walk, sending glass flying everywhere. Fearing for my children I jumped up and grabbed them, rushing for the house. They were OK, but I cried for days thinking that someone was willing to endanger two babies just for the chance to humiliate me.

"Anyone who is, or who has ever been fat has a heart full of stories: some dramatic, others less so, but all painful. Overheard comments, stares, the person who looks with a critical eye into your shopping basket as they pass you in the grocery store—it's like dying from a thousand knife cuts. No one of them is fatal, but cumulatively, they tear your heart to shreds.

"Let me add, though, that I had an epiphany several years ago. I rarely deal with this anymore. When I pass people in public, whether it's someone in the supermarket, or a group of teenagers at the mall, I make eye contact and smile and say 'hi.' I do not lower my head and try to sneak past. If I notice someone staring, I'll look them in the eye and say 'hi—how are you this morning?' I have become an in-your-face kind of activist. I do not return rudeness for rudeness, but I try for the preemptive strike of friendly, open human contact. It's not infallible, but it has made a huge difference. I approach people with an attitude of expectation that I will be treated with respect, and often, I am rewarded.

"I am very much aware that not all fat people are as defiant as I am. Not all of us have come to the place where we can look people in the eye and expect to be treated like any other person on the planet.

"I speak from experience when I tell you that many of us—maybe even most of us—are so battered by the day-to-day struggles that we become participants in our own abuse at the hands of society. I can compare it only with the mindset of an abused wife. When you've heard it often enough you start to believe it. 'Yes, you're right that I need to push myself away from the table. Yes, of course if I were only stronger. Yes, I know I'm repulsive and unworthy. God no, I'd never wear *that* in public—people would see how ugly my body is. Sure, I'll submit to surgery that amounts to medically induced bulimia. Will I lose weight? Where do I sign up? No, it's OK: My seatbelt doesn't fit, but I'll be fine without one. No, please, I understand I don't fit your company's image. Yes I'm weak: I'm not deserving of your respect, or a comfortable seat in the theater, or a loving partner, or anything else that other people take for granted . . . I'm FAT!'

"Fat people are not jolly. They are in pain because they are objects of scorn and ridicule.

"Now, all that having been said . . . I am one of the fortunate ones. I refuse to play the game. I used to wonder when medical science would come up with the magic bullet to cure obesity. I used to long for the day that there would be some miraculous cure—something that would make me 'normal.' Now, I'm not so sure that even if it did exist, I would take it. Here's why.

"I realized that the experiences of my life both good and bad have made me who I am. Being fat was one of those things, along with other situations and events in my life that have been painful and challenging, which have shaped the woman I've become. I would not be the same person if I had not experienced what I have, lived through what I have, and survived what I have.

"It contributed to my perspectives, my values, and the qualities of intellect and heart that I value. 'Fat' may not be who I am, but it has certainly had a great effect on who I am. And today, when I look in the mirror, I can honestly say that I like the person I see—fat and all. I'm finally free."

Health at Every Size

The stories above reflect several themes that appeared again and again over the course of hundreds of interviews. Five themes in particular stood out:

➤ Few Americans—and especially very few American women—
are satisfied with the appearance of their bodies. Those who
have reached something approaching peace with their appearance have often only managed to do so after a long struggle.

➤ For many Americans, weight and weight control is a topic that
consumes enormous amounts of emotional and psychological
energy. The anxiety, pain, and genuine grief this topic elicits in
so many people's lives is astounding.

➤ The simple act of actually listening to what people have to say
about this issue exposes the absurdity of the central assumption of the war on fat: that people could lose weight if they
really wanted to.

➤ For most people, the standard prescriptions for losing weight
do not work, and indeed in a significant percentage of cases the
primary recommendation—attempting to eat fewer calories—
makes people fatter than they would be otherwise. It is amazing how difficult it is for the medical establishment to accept
the fact that encouraging people to lose weight by restricting
their caloric intake actually causes the "disease" this treatment
is supposed to cure. Furthermore, while exercise and a well-
balanced diet are clearly crucial factors in maintaining good
health, they are unlikely to lead to significant long-term weight
loss. It follows that encouraging people to engage in healthy
diet and exercise habits *for the purpose of losing weight* is likely
to be counterproductive at best.

➤ People come in all shapes and sizes. Some people are thin,
some people are of average weight, and some people are fat—
and tens of millions of Americans would remain in each of
these categories even if everyone in the nation maintained optimal eating habits and activity levels. The idea that there is
something abnormal about being of more-than-average weight
is a bit of folk wisdom that by some bizarre process has been
transmuted into a supposed medical and scientific "fact."

In sum, if we consider the life experiences of Americans today
within the context of what is now known about the relationship between body mass, eating habits, physical activity, and overall health,
we can begin to construct a saner model for understanding the link between weight and health than that reflected in the pseudoscientific or-

thodoxy of BMI tables and "ideal" weight ranges. Specifically, a growing number of obesity researchers, eating disorder specialists, nutritionists, dieticians, and others who have come to reject the basic tenets of
the war against fat are constructing an alternative paradigm for dealing
with the relationship between weight and health, that is coming to be
known as the Health at Every Size movement, or HAES.

One of the leading proponents of HAES is Joanne Ikeda, a researcher in the University of California-Berkeley's Department of Nutritional Science. Ikeda points out that, in the wake of what she calls
"the disintegration of the traditional medical paradigm" for dealing
with persons of more than average weight (i.e., advising such people to
diet and exercise *in order to lose weight*), a new model is beginning to
emerge—one "based on the belief that although we may not be able
to help fat people permanently lose weight, we can help them improve
their health and reduce their risk for chronic disease." The HAES
movement builds on the insight that perhaps the single most crucial
misconception feeding America's obsession with fat is the notion that
people of the same height who eat normally and engage in an optimal
level of physical activity will all maintain roughly the same weight.
This idea is implicit in the federal government's declaration that a
"healthy" body weight is one that translates into a BMI of between
18.5 and 24.9. (According to this formula, a healthy weight for a woman
of average height must be somewhere between 108 and 144 pounds.)

As we have seen, there is no credible scientific basis for this assertion. Taken as a whole, the medical literature simply does not support
the proposition that women of average height who weigh 157 or 177 or
207 pounds will be less healthy or have a lower life expectancy than
women who weigh 117 pounds, assuming that all these women engage in healthy eating habits and regular physical activity (the larger
women will have, on average, much better health than the thinner
ones if the former are physically active while the latter are sedentary).
The myth at the center of the war on fat is a person cannot have a
healthy lifestyle and yet still weigh 25 or 50 or even 100 pounds more
than the cultural ideal. HAES proponents point out that people who
engage in normal, healthy eating—that is, people who eat a balanced
diet, who generally eat in response to hunger, and normally stop eating
when sated—and who are also physically active, vary enormously in
weight, as do people with poor diets and sedentary lifestyles. HAES
proponents also emphasize that the size of someone's body rarely tells

you anything about whether he or she has a healthy lifestyle. In Ikeda's words, "there is no ideal body size, shape, or weight that every individual should strive to achieve."

The HAES movement itself is based on three core principles, all derived from a comprehensive interpretation of the extant medical literature on weight and health. These principles are outlined by Jon Robison, professor at Michigan State University and coeditor of the medical journal, *Health at Every Size*, as follows:

1. The claims that more-than-average weight causes poor health and premature death, and that weight loss leads to improved health are not supported by the medical literature.

2. Weight loss is not at present a sustainable outcome for the vast majority of people.

3. There is considerable evidence that promoting weight loss does more harm than good.

One of the HAES movement's goals is to help medical professionals become more aware of what the medical literature on weight and weight loss actually indicates. For instance, HAES proponents aim to publicize medical studies demonstrating that people who ingest exactly the same number of calories and engage in identical levels of physical activity end up gaining or losing vastly different amounts of weight. A classic example is provided by a 1990 *New England Journal of Medicine* study that involved overfeeding twelve sets of identical twins 1,000 extra calories per day, six days per week, while the subjects maintained substantially identical levels of physical activity. (The subjects lived in dormitories, and their activities were monitored twenty-four hours per day.) After just seven weeks, the resulting weight gain among these twenty-four men varied by 300%, from 9 pounds to almost 30 pounds. The variation between sets of twins was much larger than within sets, which indicates the strong role genetics plays in this matter.

Similarly, a 1999 study published in *Science* overfed sixteen subjects 1,000 calories per day for eight weeks. As might be expected, the bodies of the subjects reacted to this overfeeding by increasing energy expenditure. (This is an example of the famous "set point" theory, that predicts that the body's metabolism will change in reaction to either caloric scarcity or caloric overload, in an attempt to maintain body weight.) The most striking finding that came out of this study was the radically different amounts of energy expended by the study's subjects through what is known as "activity thermogenesis," especially non-exercise activity thermogenesis (NEAT). NEAT is largely determined by activities of daily living, such as fidgeting, maintaining posture, spontaneous muscle contraction, and the like—things most people do not keep track of, and often are not even aware of. The change in NEAT brought on by the overfeeding of these sixteen subjects ranged from essentially nothing to 692 calories *per day*. Six hundred and ninety-two calories is about what the average runner will expend in the course of a ten-kilometer (6.2-mile) race. In other words, even within this tiny sample, the metabolic reactions of the subjects' bodies to excess calories varied by several orders of magnitude. As obesity researcher and HAES proponent Glenn Gaesser points out, "with this much variation demonstrated in studies involving a handful of individuals, imagine the variation you might find among 285,000,000 Americans, or the six billion members of the human race. BMI charts are much simpler."

The HAES movement advocates a reshaping of medical practice in regard to "overweight" and "obesity" that would encourage medical professionals to focus on what is most important to the health of people of all shapes and sizes: being or becoming physically active, engaging in healthful eating (that is, eating a nutritious, well-balanced mix of foods in response to internal body cues, rather than attempting to reduce caloric intake in response to externally imposed rules), and accepting not merely the inevitability, but the positive desirability of the diverse forms healthy human bodies take. The movement's seven "principles for medical practice" are: A healthy weight is the weight a person maintains while living a healthy life; overweight (BMI 25 to 29.9) is not an independent cause of morbidity and mortality; thinner is not necessarily healthier; the health risks associated with obesity (BMI 30+) are exaggerated; permanent weight loss is out of reach for most people; improved health is within the reach of almost everyone; and weight prejudice is both unreasonable and unnecessary.

HAES, then, recognizes that it is both normal and desirable for people's bodies to vary across a far larger range than the narrow spectrum of "ideal" weight recommended by the weight loss industry and its allies in the medical and public health establishment. Assuming that everyone either can or should maintain a BMI of between 18.5 and 24.9 ignores everything we know about human genetic and cultural diversity. As Glenn Gaesser points out, "the genetic component of our fat makeup is, so far as we know, unalterable. If one person is genetically programmed to have twice the number of fat cells that someone else does, then it can only be expected that the first person will have a set point for body fat, and body weight, that is much higher than the second person's. For millions this higher set point has resulted in weights that are above height-weight table recommendations. They are not inherently less healthy than other people, just *inherently heavier*."

Indeed, in the wake of decades of failed attempts to make larger people thin, medical researchers are finally beginning to test approaches to dealing with higher-than-average weight that focus on something other than promoting weight loss. The initial results of this research are striking. For example, Linda Bacon, a nutrition researcher at the University of California-Davis, has just completed a two-year clinical trial in which two groups of "obese" women participated in, respectively, a traditional diet and weight loss program, and a HAES program. The former program was focused on changing nutritional and exercise habits to promote weight loss; the latter also aimed to improve nutritional and exercise habits, but in addition strove to promote body acceptance and self-acceptance generally. The HAES program therefore eschewed weight loss as a goal, and instead tried to help participants disentangle feelings of self-worth from their weight. In particular, it focused on getting the participants to regulate their eating on the basis of internal body cues, as opposed to external rules, and on helping participants become more active, by finding activities that allowed them to enjoy their bodies, without regard to whether these activities resulted in any weight loss.

Initially, the health of both groups enjoyed comparable improvement as measured by blood pressure, LDL cholesterol, energy expenditure, evidence of eating disorders, body dissatisfaction, depression, and self-esteem. The traditional diet-and-exercise group lost weight; the HAES group did not. After two years, the subjects following the traditional program had regained almost all their lost weight (indeed, given that nearly half of them dropped out of the study, it seems likely that the diet group maintained no net weight loss, and may have gained weight. By contrast, almost none of the HAES subjects dropped out). But the study's most striking finding was that, while the diet group sustained none of the health improvements it experienced initially, the HAES group sustained all of them! Studies of this sort suggest both that the medical profession's traditional focus on weight loss is hazardous to physiological and psychological health, and that the key to improving the health of larger-than-average persons is to focus on appropriate lifestyle changes while promoting body acceptance, rather than continuing the futile quest to make fat people thin.

The two most important points to take away from the HAES message is that, subject to a few exceptions at the statistical extremes, there is no way to tell whether a person is at a healthy weight merely by determining that person's body mass, and that body weight in and of itself is almost never relevant to good health. People who engage in healthful eating and who are at least moderately physically active will have better health, on average, than those who don't, and thus the question of whether a person is thin, fat, or somewhere in between is largely irrelevant to evaluating his or her health.

Or to put it another way, when people are "abnormally" fat or "abnormally" thin, the problem is not fatness or thinness per se: it is that body mass *in these particular cases* is an indicator of unhealthy eating habits and/or inadequate levels of physical activity. Many other people will have exactly the same body mass as these individuals, and yet their fatness or thinness does not indicate similar problems— because their fatness or thinness is not in any sense abnormal. Until one determines whether an individual actually engages in unhealthy habits such as compulsive dieting, binge eating, or a sedentary lifestyle, it is at best meaningless and at worst destructive to label him or her "too fat" or "too thin."

Consider the HAES message in the context of the narratives that made up the first part of this chapter. Joyce is almost certainly a woman who would be quite thin—a below-average-weight woman—if she ate and exercised normally, who has become anorexic as a consequence of cultural pressures that have given her a distorted sense of what "normal" means. Perhaps the most frustrating aspect of the war on fat is the refusal of the health establishment to recognize that this kind of thinking—what is called "anorexic ideation"—is an inevitable product of cultural norms that damages the self-images of tens of millions of Americans who are not technically anorexic, in much the same way these same norms have harmed people like Joyce. Plenty of thin, average-weight and fat people have just as distorted a sense of what a "normal" weight is as Joyce does, and they are being damaged by that distortion in ways that are more subtle, but not necessarily less serious, than the ways anorexic thinking damages those who have been formally diagnosed with eating disorders.

Elaine, for example, might be classified as either normally or abnormally thin: at 5'9" and a weight in the 130s, she is of considerably less-than-average weight. She eats normally and gets far more than enough exercise to maintain good health. Given that she runs sixty miles per week, it's probable that she would be of a more average weight if she exercised moderately; still, from the perspective of physical health, a person who maintains something akin to a normally thin build by eating normally and exercising intensely is someone who is dealing with weight issues in a far more constructive way than dieters and other abnormal eaters. Nevertheless, Elaine, like so many of the people I interviewed, is haunted by fears of becoming fat, and spent much of her youth subject to the intermittent conviction that she was fat, despite all the evidence to the contrary.

This conviction, along with the effects of dieting, eventually managed to make her much fatter than she ever would have become in a society with a saner attitude toward weight. Her ability to find her way back to a world of relatively normal eating is a tribute to her psychological strength; but comments such as that she "doesn't really like food" indicate that journey has come at a considerable cost. She, too, has found it difficult to hold on to what "normal" means in the context of weight, body image, and health.

Sarah, on the other hand, appears to be of average weight (absurdly, our federal government would categorize her as "overweight"). She is not a dieter, but she, too, probably maintains a somewhat lower weight than the natural weight she would carry if she continued to eat normally but exercised only moderately. Sarah's situation is also a testament to the arbitrariness of our present ideal of female beauty: In most cultures at most times, her figure would have been considered ideal; yet in America today, the mere fact that she looks like a woman is enough to make her unhappiness about her body the major source of anxiety in her life.

Michael and Cynthia are normally fat persons—or rather they would be normally fat, if decades of dieting had not made them considerably fatter than they would have been otherwise. Both of these remarkably intelligent and eloquent individuals have suffered the effects of growing up in a culture that seems incapable of grasping the simple truth that some people are destined to be fat, just as others are destined to be tall or short or freckled or curly-haired. Their ultimately successful struggle to reject the endless bombardment of propaganda and outright lies about "excess" weight to which people such as themselves are subjected has a genuinely heroic quality.

As for Julia and Rachel, their stories capture the essence of why we need to reject the lies at the core of the war on fat. Unfortunately a simple narration cannot capture much of the passion and pain that these talented young women, already accomplished and full of promise, conveyed when they described what they had endured in the course of struggling with these issues. The confession at the end of Julia's narrative, and Rachel's words about having lost so much to the power of this demon we unleash on ourselves, continue to haunt me. (A colleague and friend of Rachel's who knows something of her past told me, "The shocking thing is that Rachel is one of the sanest, most together people I know. If this can happen to her, it can happen to anyone.")

At such moments, I find myself thinking of my nine-year-old daughter. It is difficult to convey the depth of the anger I feel at the thought that she seems bound to suffer the consequences of living in a culture that will fixate on the idiotic notion that her body isn't what it "should" be, simply because she is not genetically predisposed to be extremely thin. It is true that this is not the worst form of oppression in the world. But make no mistake: It is a form of oppression—one that causes a vast amount of unnecessary suffering. And let us not lose sight of just who the chief architects of that oppression are: those who both encourage and profit from the depraved idea that the greatest accomplishment to which my daughter can aspire is to give herself over to the kind of destructive obsession that might one day allow her to move from a size 12 to a size 6 dress.

PART III

FAT POLITICS

Early in my first term, I used to go jogging before seven in the morning, and the White House press would inexplicably cover me. I mean, what is there to cover? An aging, overweight man puffing along at a quarter to seven along the highway? They thought I would drop dead of a heart attack or something.

—BILL CLINTON, APRIL 2002

15

The Feeding of the President

EARLY IN 1994, Hillary Rodham Clinton made a little-noted but fateful decision: She decided her husband needed to lose weight. This decision was in part a reaction to the seemingly endless series of fat jokes that had marked the first year of the Clinton presidency. Who could forget the *Saturday Night Live* sketch in which Clinton went on a jog with his Secret Service agents, which lasted about two hundred yards before detouring into a McDonald's? Once inside, Bill gobbled up cheeseburgers and fries belonging to bemused customers, while using the rapidly disappearing food items as props for an impromptu speech about Somali warlords. Clinton was often photographed jogging, and wisecracks about his flabby thighs and jiggling belly became staples for Jay Leno and David Letterman, as well as for dozens of less famous comedians from coast to coast.

Indeed, while Clinton was hardly fat, the fact that he was, by late 1993, perhaps 30 pounds heavier than the cultural ideal for a man of his height and social position became the basis for what is called a synecdoche, a figure of speech in which a less inclusive term is used to stand for a broader set of characteristics. To call attention to Clinton's weight—to label him fat—became a kind of shorthand for everything about the man that seemed most disturbing: his lack of personal discipline, his self-indulgence, his aura of immaturity, and most of all his reckless sensuality, especially the sort of out-of-control philandering that led to the famous "bimbo eruptions" that nearly sank his 1992 presidential campaign. From the first days of his presidency, Bill Clinton's purported weight problem became the easiest—and therefore the most common—way of referencing the metaphorical figure of Slick Willie: the corpulent good ol' boy whose plump frame became a faintly ludicrous visual cue, reminding those who laughed at the sight of it of their suspicion that, underneath a layer of easygoing fat, Clinton might well lack the steely core of self-discipline required of anyone occupying the most powerful office in the world.

Thus, in retrospect, it should have come as no surprise that his wife, who for obvious reasons was exquisitely sensitive to this set of perceptions regarding her husband's weaknesses, should have taken decisive steps to do something about her husband's politically problematic waistline. When they moved into the White House the Clintons inherited French-trained chef Pierre Chambrin from the first Bush administration, and for more than a year Chambrin feted his most famous client with many of the classic dishes of the Gallic kitchen. Then, in early 1994, Hillary fired him. Three years later Chambrin revealed that he believed the first lady got rid of him because he was too fat and had a French accent. "I think the reason they didn't want me is because, even if I have been an American since 1977, I didn't fit the profile of the chef of the White House, because of my accent and the fact that I'm overweight," Chambrin said in 1997.

Chambrin's story came to light in the context of a lawsuit by another fired Clinton employee, whose lawyers deposed the deposed chef, thus forcing him to break a vow of silence he had taken about the whole matter, a vow he took in return for a generous severance package and a good recommendation. White House officials denied Chambrin's charges, of course. According to Clinton's people, Chambrin was fired not because he was fat, but because his cooking was making the president fat. Naturally they didn't phrase the matter in exactly those terms: The White House claimed Chambrin was let go as a consequence of "a desire for lighter, American cuisine for the first family." Specifically, a spokeswoman for Hillary Clinton claimed Mrs. Clinton wanted to shift the White House's daily menu from the butter and demi-glacé that dominates classic French cuisine to "a more American style with heart-healthy ingredients." It was strictly a question of health, you see.

Anyway, Chambrin was replaced by American chef Walter Scheib, who specializes in low-fat cooking. (By the way, it's true that the French eat a much higher-fat diet than Americans. They are also a good deal thinner, on average.) Suddenly the president was finding skinless chicken breasts and steamed broccoli on his plate instead of goose liver pâté and escargot wrapped in bacon. And, coincidentally or not, he began to lose weight. Although precise information regarding presidential weights remains a closely guarded state secret, the photographic record is clear: Between mid-1994 and early 1996, Bill Clinton lost somewhere in the neighborhood of 25 to 30 pounds.

One evening toward the end of this time, a White House intern named Monica Lewinsky took a couple of slices of vegetarian pizza into the Oval Office. The rest, as they say, is history—the kind of bizarre history that could only have taken place in the food-obsessed world of contemporary America, but history nevertheless. To truly understand that history, we must understand how matters of personal appearance in general, and of fat in particular, have played a key role in the lives of the principal players in the Lewinsky affair.

The following passage is from *Purposes of the Heart*, a transparent roman à clef written by a high school classmate of Bill Clinton's, Dolly Kyle Browning. The book is centered around an off-and-on affair between Kelly, a character whose life story is basically identical to the author's, and Cameron Coulter, who bears an uncanny resemblance to Bill Clinton. The quoted passage takes place when Kelly, who has gone to the airport to serve as Cameron's driver for the day, is shocked by the physical appearance of Mallory Cheatham, the woman whom Cameron introduces as his fiancée.

> The dowdy-looking woman stepped up beside him and Kelly realized that she was of their generation, not middle-aged as her first glance indicated. Kelly wondered why Cameron would haul such a person in the plane with him in public. She was wearing a misshapen brown dress that must have been intended to hide her lumpy body. The garment was long, but stopped too soon to hide her fat ankles and thick calves which, to Kelly's amazement, were covered with black hair. Thick brown sandals did nothing to conceal her wide feet and the hair on her toes . . . [Her] eyes bulged out of focus behind Coke-bottle thick lenses in dark, heavy frames, competing with the dark, thick eyebrow which crossed from one side of her

forehead to the other . . . She noticed that the woman emitted
a definite odor of perspiration and greasy hair. Kelly's heart
went out to the poor creature.

"Mallory Cheatham" is of course Hillary Rodham. Exaggerated as
Browning's description no doubt is, it captures the effect that their
first encounters with Hillary had on many of Bill's Arkansas friends,
particularly women. Indeed, a woman of considerably greater importance in Bill Clinton's life than Dolly Browning shared Browning's low
opinion of the public figure presented by Bill's intended. Virginia
Dwire, as Bill's mother was then known, was appalled by Hillary's willingness to flout the conventions of Hot Springs, Arkansas, where no
self-respecting lady would dare appear in public without spending a
good deal of time in front of the makeup mirror first. (In a touch
straight out of Faulkner, the only person in Bill's immediate family who
tried to make his fiancée feel welcome was Virginia's new husband Jeff
Dwire, a hairdresser who favored diamond pinkie rings, and who had
done time in federal prison for fraud. At the time of Hillary's first visit
to Arkansas, Dwire ran a salon patronized by the prostitutes of a local
madam named Maxine. His wife, however, still considered the dowdy
alumna of Wellesley and Yale Law School not good enough for her ambitious son.)

Bill Clinton told his family in no uncertain terms that they had
better get used to having Hillary around: "Look, I want you to know
that I've had it up to *here* with beauty queens. I have to have somebody
I can talk with." Nevertheless, Hillary Rodham knew full well that if
she was going to marry Bill Clinton, she had to prepare to be the wife
of an Arkansas politician, and quite possibly of the state's future governor. Gradually, she began to shed the outward trappings of 1960s-style
upper-class bohemia. Indeed, photographs of her taken at the time of
Bill's initial election to the governorship in 1978 captured the image of
a woman whose appearance now bore no resemblance to the radical
manqué look Hillary favored in college and law school. Glowing with
wifely pride, Hillary, who at the time was not yet thirty, looked like a
matron out of a Vermeer canvas, her round cheeks framed by a conservative bun of brown hair. These photographs make it clear that she
was a woman who seemed destined for a plump middle age: Like her
husband, Hillary is basically an endomorph, and therefore prone to
put on weight unless she takes fanatical steps to maintain something

approaching a fashionably thin figure. Needless to say, over the years during which her husband rose to public prominence, she took those steps.

A woman who has known Hillary for more than three decades, and who worked closely with her at one time, told me that the future first lady made a conscious decision in the late 1970s to lose weight and keep it off. "Of course if there was ever anybody you could predict would manage to stay slim despite everything, it would be Hillary Rodham," she says. "She's the strongest-willed, most disciplined person I've ever known." Others close to Hillary confirm that for many years she has battled successfully to maintain a figure far slimmer than the one heredity and environment intended her to have. "It's all part of the same thing that made her change her hairstyle every few weeks during their first term," a former White House aide told me. "She's very sensitive to remarks about her appearance—and who wouldn't be, given how vicious some of those remarks have been."

Still, compared to those of her husband, Hillary's weight anxieties have remained relatively muted. Several people who know Bill Clinton well have commented, on and off the record, about how the experience of growing up a fat kid has shaped his self-perception, and indeed has played an important part in producing the underlying motivations that have fueled his reckless behavior toward women. For example, when he was first elected governor, his philandering became so brazen that it was soon a semipublic topic throughout Arkansas political circles. Long-time friend Susan McDougal recalls Clinton telling her at the time, "This is fun. Women are throwing themselves at me. All the while I was growing up, I was the fat boy in Big Boy jeans." (It's worth noting in this context that Bill's mother divorced Roger Clinton in 1962, when Bill was fifteen, only to remarry Roger later that year after Bill's stepfather lost 35 pounds.)

Along similar lines, a lawyer and lobbyist who has known Clinton for many years told me that Clinton asked her "on more than one occasion" if a particular piece of clothing "made him look fat." "I guess I more or less assumed he was joking, but I couldn't really tell for sure," she says. "It struck me as odd, though—it's the kind of thing women friends ask each other all the time, but coming from him it just seemed rather strange."

Clinton's interest in the topic of weight, whether his own or that of others, has been amply documented by Monica Lewinsky. She told

Andrew Morton that, on the occasion of their first tryst in the Oval Office, Monica found Bill's anxieties about his weight so similar to her own that they helped endear him to her: "It was such a sweet moment. It was the first time I had seen him without a shirt, and he sucked in his stomach. I thought it was the cutest thing. I said, 'Oh, you don't have to do that—I like your tummy.' It was very endearing and sweet—it made him seem more like a real person to me." Similarly, on one occasion when Monica addressed Bill by her pet name for him, "Handsome," Clinton replied to the effect that, "You may think of me as handsome, but when I look in the mirror I see a fat boy who can't shoot a basketball."

Monica's appreciation of Clinton's exquisite sensitivity to weight issues was further enhanced by the fact that he never failed to compliment her for looking slim, whenever she lost even a little weight, or wore something that flattered her figure, or if he merely wanted to comfort her at a time of stress. "I saw you in the hall today—you looked really skinny," was a typical comment, one that, in some form or another, Bill made to Monica numerous times over the months of their affair.

In doing so, Clinton displayed his famous ability to hone in on the precise issue that was of most importance to his audience. To say that Monica Lewinsky was and is obsessed with her weight is an understatement, even taking into account that she is a product of a cultural context (upper-class Los Angeles in the 1980s and 1990s) in which weight obsession is very much the norm among women of her generation. Among the sixty-odd topics indexed under her name in Andrew Morton's tell-all biography, *Monica's Story*, "weight" garners more entries than all but one; and indeed the book, written with Monica's full cooperation, is in many ways a testament to the centrality of weight issues in her life.

Monica's teenage years were dominated by the devastation being a "fat" girl at Beverly Hills High wrought to her self-esteem: "A 'normal' high school girl," she thought, "was thin, a cheerleader, had lots of boyfriends and went to endless parties. That wasn't me. Everybody looked great, everyone was very conscious of how they looked there and so being overweight was not acceptable. The pressure was horrid." She became miserable and depressed, her grades suffered, and, in a reaction typical of the time and place, her mother decided her daughter had an eating disorder. Marcia Lewinsky wanted to send Monica to a famous weight loss program in North Carolina that allows its in-mates to eat only rice for an entire month, in a bid to get them to lose 30 pounds in as many days. Luckily, this dangerous bit of quackery was vetoed by Monica's father, but the very idea that a mother would be willing to put her daughter on a medically insane starvation diet simply because she had an inappropriate body type for the social scene at Beverly Hills High School speaks volumes regarding how un-hinged the cultural milieu in which Monica grew up was in regard to questions of weight.

In any case, at the end of her junior year in high school Monica ended up going to see a therapist and joining Overeaters Anonymous. Thus began a classic pattern of yo-yo dieting that seems to have lasted to this day, more than a decade later. Monica's weight has fluctuated by more than 40 pounds several times during this period, but what has remained constant is her persistent sense of low self-esteem. One of her best friends, Catherine Davis, sees Monica's poor self-image as the key to understanding why she keeps getting romantically involved with manipulative married men: "Her relationship with Andy [Blieler] was damaging to her in the same way as her affair with the President. She was involving herself with a man who was never going to be hers and it was stopping her from being a normal woman going on normal dates. In some ways she thought she wasn't good enough to be loved."

Another friend remembers her first serious conversation with Monica: A two-hour talk in a parking lot, during which Monica talked mostly about how her inability to maintain weight loss was the major source of unhappiness in her life. Andrew Morton interprets her assumption—on the occasion of her first kiss from Bill Clinton—that his regular girlfriend was temporarily absent from the White House, as a sign that "she always saw herself as second best in her relationships with men. Just as at school and at college, at the White House she as-sumed that any man who took the slightest interest in her did so out of pity or because there was no one else available." Many of Monica's re-marks to Morton support this view. "Normally," she told him, "when I get ready to go to a hoity-toity event I become a basket case, down on myself, thinking that I look fat and ugly in everything." It's hardly sur-prising that, after having internalized the destructive message that there is something terribly wrong with a woman of average height who weighs 150 pounds, Monica proved to be vulnerable to the manipula-tive schemes of unscrupulous men—and those of one woman.

In retrospect, it makes perfect sense that what brought Monica Lewinsky and Linda Tripp together was a shared bond of misery about their respective appearances. Twenty years older than Monica, Tripp had been teased mercilessly as a teenage girl growing up in New Jersey in the 1960s. Tall, gawky, and broad-shouldered, her classmates called her "Gus," after the NBA star Gus Johnson. By the time Tripp met Monica Lewinsky in the summer of 1996, she was a bitter middle-aged woman, dealing with the aftermath of the collapse of her twenty-year marriage, and her involuntary transfer from a job at the White House to the Pentagon, to which, for very different reasons, Lewinsky had also been exiled. Morton relates that the two women at first "shared diet tips, [and] in the course of a year Monica encourag[ed] her new friend to lose sixty pounds, and offer[ed] her enthusiastic approval when Tripp joined Weight Watchers."

Something else that has become clear in hindsight is that Tripp was obsessed with Bill Clinton, and that she suspected from the first the existence of some sort of romantic entanglement between Monica and the president. Indeed, it went beyond that: Tripp, who liked to boast that Hillary Clinton was jealous of her because she suspected Tripp was having an affair with Bill, soon began to live out some strange psychic fantasy life through Monica. (For example, she refused to meet Monica's mother Marcia until Tripp herself had lost weight.) Morton, plausibly enough, interprets this sort of behavior as evidence that Tripp was stalking Monica, "not physically, but [by] attempting to invade her psyche." Tripp, it seems, saw Monica as someone through whom she could seduce Bill Clinton by proxy, as a prelude to destroying the man Tripp both desired and despised. For months, she deviously suggested over and over again to her new friend that Monica would be able to return to the White House after the November 1996 election, and that "she [Monica] was just the girl for the president."

These manipulative suggestions bore fruit, when, depressed after Clinton failed to contact her in the days after his reelection, Monica finally confided her secret—that she had been conducting an on-and-off affair with Clinton for nearly a year. An exultant Tripp then began to concoct a scheme that would pay back the Clinton administration for the mistreatment to which she believed she had been subjected, and would also make her rich and famous in the bargain. She spent the next months cultivating her friendship with Lewinsky, while planning simultaneously to betray her friend in a tell-all book, which would consist of whatever combination of facts and rumors about the sordid side of the Clinton administration she had managed to collect over the course of the previous four years. Monica's affair with the president would, of course, be the centerpiece of this projected text. Still, Tripp knew her scheme lacked one crucial element: Some piece of independent corroborating evidence that would hold up in the face of any denials Monica might issue when her supposed friend finally sprang her long-prepared trap. (And indeed, Morton reveals that Monica's contingency plan to deal with any revelations was to deny everything, and if necessary to go so far as to claim she had fabricated the whole story about an affair with the president.)

It was at this juncture, in the fall of 1997, that the weight obsessions of two of the principal actors in the scandal played their most direct role in bringing about the eventual impeachment of the president of the United States. Encouraged by Monica, Tripp had spent the previous months on a strict diet, and had lost a good deal of weight. In order to congratulate her friend, Monica invited Linda to examine the contents of her "fat closet"—that part of her wardrobe made up of clothes Monica was either too fat or too thin to wear at whatever point she was currently occupying on the classic yo-yo dieting curve—so that Linda might pick out one of Monica's larger dresses, into which she (Tripp) could now fit. And it was during this ritual—a fairly common one among friends whose friendship is based on their mutual attempts to lose weight—that Monica revealed to her friend the existence of the infamous semen-stained blue dress. Far from keeping the dress as some sort of protective evidence or fetishistic trophy, Monica had simply neglected to have it dry-cleaned because she hadn't been able to fit into it for several months, and, being chronically short of money, she saw no need to do so until she lost enough weight to be able to wear it again. Instantly, Tripp knew she had found the corroborative evidence she needed.

Almost immediately afterward, Tripp began taping her phone conversations with Monica. When, a few weeks after the visit to the fat closet, Monica told Tripp that she had finally lost enough weight to wear the dress to her father's family's Thanksgiving dinner—an occasion fraught with anxiety for Monica because her female cousins were all slender—Tripp began to panic. In a phone conversation she recorded for what turned out to be a Nixonian posterity, Tripp urgently cautioned Monica not to clean the dress: "Now, all I would say to you is, you have a very long life ahead of you, and I don't know what's going to happen to you. Neither do you. I would rather you had that in your possession if you need it years from now."

Unconvinced, Monica told her friend that she planned to wear it anyhow: After all, it was one of her most slimming outfits. A desperate Tripp then played her trump card, telling Monica bluntly that the dress made her look fat. Predictably, this tack worked more successfully on Monica's ever-fragile psyche, and she decided not to have the dress cleaned after all. At this point Linda Tripp realized that she could not delay her scheme much longer, and, after a farcical attempt to steal the dress failed, the elaborate perjury trap she had helped Bill Clinton's most rabid political enemies prepare was finally sprung, in the course of the president's deposition in the Paula Jones case.

What does the Lewinsky scandal tell us about the effects fear and loathing of fat can have in American life today? Ultimately, a great deal. Beginning at the simplest level of causation, if Monica Lewinsky had not been transformed into a yo-yo dieter by her experiences at Beverly Hills High, there would have been no semen-stained dress hiding in a fat closet—and without the existence of that dress it is extremely unlikely that the scandal, if it had existed at all, would ever have risen above the level of something like the Katherine Willey affair. But the causal chain that links our culture's obsession with fat and the impeachment of the forty-second president of the United States is far more complicated and interesting than that.

For one thing, fat brought Monica Lewinsky and Linda Tripp together. Their shared anxiety about fat formed the basis of their friendship, and was perhaps their single most common topic of conversation. Indeed, the power of the bond that can be created by a mutual weight obsession is evidenced by the fact that Linda Tripp—a woman of an entirely different generation who had almost nothing else in common with Monica—became a close enough friend to be trusted with a secret that Monica knew would have devastating consequences to both her and many others if it were ever revealed.

Moreover, fat prejudice and fat phobia battered Monica's self-esteem to the point where, rather than dating men with whom she might be able to develop a healthy long-term relationship, she sought out serial adulterers such as Clinton and Andy Bleiler, whose manipulative and callous treatment of her confirmed the feelings of self-hatred a society obsessed with thinness had taught Monica to internalize.

The media's reaction to Monica Lewinsky illustrated many of the ugliest features of that obsession. Consider the implications of the fact that a computer database search for the year 1998 turns up more than one hundred news stories that feature both the words "Monica Lewin-sky" and "zaftig." (In a symptomatic instance of semantic drift, "zaftig," a German-Yiddish word that literally means "juicy," has over the course of the past century gone from being a term used to describe an erotically curvaceous woman to becoming an increasingly nasty euphemism for "fat.") At one point, a significant percentage of the news stories about Monica were making some sort of snide reference to her weight, while the more gossipy tabloids, unconstrained by the mores of supposedly objective journalism, were often nothing less than sadistic: "A fat cheesy slut" was one particularly vicious description employed in the headline of a national magazine.

In fact, Monica's sexual recklessness was characteristic of that often found among women with particularly poor body images, as they desperately seek evidence they possess an attractiveness to men that the culture reminds them dozens of times a day is supposedly reserved for the sorts of extraordinarily thin women they can never become. Indeed, in an odd way Monica herself became a comforting figure to many women, if only because she confirmed the sexual power a traditionally curvaceous pulchritude can wield over the most powerful men, even (or perhaps especially?) when, as more than one woman whom I interviewed put it, the woman who wields that power "doesn't look like a model."

To that part of the culture that harbors an irrational fear and loathing of fat, however, the fact that the president of the United States had an affair with a "fat" Jewish girl from Beverly Hills represented something quite different. Although never stated explicitly, the subtext of many of the stories about the "zaftig" intern was fairly clear: Monica Lewinsky embodied, at a deep level of social anxiety, a sort of reincarnation of the rapacious, sexually insatiable Jewess of European lore. Much like Bill Clinton's "fatness," Monica's curvaceous physique became and has remained a metaphor for everything about the cultural symbolism of fat that disturbs America's self-denying (and increasingly famished) elites.

Similarly, whatever else Bill Clinton's own self-destructive promiscuity may involve, it can in part be understood as a classic symptom of the grown man who has never gotten over being the fat kid who couldn't shoot a basketball. Just as the woman whose insecurities he exploited was incapable of believing that a man could consider her something other than a substitute for a more desirable woman, Clinton seems never to have gotten over the puerile thrill he first experienced when, as he told Susan McDougal, he discovered that women would "throw themselves" at him when he achieved a sufficiently powerful political position. Indeed, rather than bearing the marks of the coldly calculating sensualist, Clinton's reckless behavior illustrates the compulsive pattern of sexual adventurism of a man who can never quite find the unimpeachable affirmation of desirability he needs in order to believe he is no longer the fat boy in Big Boy jeans.

Despite all this, Clinton did his best—according to Dick Morris and others—to be "good" during the 1992 presidential campaign and throughout the first two years of his presidency. In this regard it's significant that even the indefatigable Ken Starr was unable to dig up any evidence of sexual misbehavior during this time, which perhaps not coincidentally was the only period during Clinton's presidency when he was eating exactly what he wanted to eat on a regular basis. One doesn't need to subscribe to a crude hydraulic theory of the id to acknowledge that a man who is given free rein over some of his deepest sensual desires will in all likelihood find it easier to rein in some others. Yet in America today we've created a political and cultural climate that doesn't allow the president of the nation to smoke, drink, or get fat. Given this, it shouldn't exactly come as a shock that a man like Bill Clinton eventually reverted to other habits that could be more easily hidden.

As distasteful as it is to recount the sexual details of the Clinton-Lewinsky affair, those details are quite revelatory in regard to the ultimate connection between fat anxiety and the impeachment of the president. Thanks to the intrepid labors of Judge Starr, all of America was made aware that Bill Clinton never actually engaged in sexual intercourse with Monica Lewinsky. *Monica's Story* tells us that in fact he flatly refused to do so when Monica tried to pressure him to consummate their relationship in the traditional fashion. Monica herself interpreted this as a coolly rational decision on the president's part not to incur the extra risks that such a consummation would entail, but other interpretations are certainly possible.

Indeed it is possible to see a basic parallel between Clinton's sexual transgressions with Monica Lewinsky and the furtive cheating engaged in by "bad" dieters, which of course almost all dieters eventually become. Specifically, Clinton not only refused to have intercourse with Monica: It isn't even clear from the Starr Report, despite the lurid detail into which it regularly descends, that any of the occasions on which Monica Lewinsky performed fellatio on Clinton ended with a non-masturbatory orgasm on the part of the nation's chief executive (it is clear that most of them did not). We might note that a willingness to receive sexual favors that consist of unconsummated oral sex, while refusing more satisfactory encounters, is somewhat reminiscent of the dieter who keeps slinking back into the kitchen in the middle of the night to "indulge" in a series of thin slices of an ultimately unsatisfying fat-free pound cake, instead of, for example, finishing one's dinner off with a couple of scoops of real vanilla ice cream.

Yet the cold fact of the matter is that, at this point in American history, millions of voters would consider the sight of a fat president far more disturbing than the sight of a president who argues under oath about what the meaning of the word "is" is, or who betrays a former lover by calling her "that woman" on national television. Hillary Clinton, having spent her life struggling successfully with the demons of dieting, understands this. She also understood it in 1994, when she decided it was crucial to her husband's presidency for him to lose weight. She knew that a fat Bill Clinton would strike too many influential people as an image out of some sort of trailer trash Camelot, and so she took characteristically aggressive steps to ensure that the feeding of the president didn't produce the sort of thick-necked good ol' boy that her husband's genes and upbringing had so strongly predisposed him to become.

Similarly, the same social dynamic that, as we shall see in the next chapter, made law professor and political commentator Susan Estrich's mother so determined that her daughter would not return "fat," for her sophomore year at Hillary Clinton's alma mater also ensured that Marcia Lewinsky would attempt, two decades later, to send her daughter to a month-long inpatient program that would quite literally starve her down to a socially acceptable weight. These are merely two examples of how, for many upwardly mobile Jewish families, fatness represents what it also represents to, among others, ambitious small-town Southern politicians, and professional-class members of ethnic minorities: the most visible and therefore unacceptable sign that you are still on the outside looking in. (In her diet book *Making the Case for Yourself,* Estrich describes what to her is clearly a disturbing sight: "My neighborhood is full of Orthodox Jewish women with four children and forty extra pounds.") Indeed, to be fat—or rather what is considered fat—in America today has to a significant extent both replaced and overlapped the traditional social significance once ascribed to being black, or Jewish, or "white trash."

This, then, is the moral of the sad tale of Bill Clinton and Monica Lewinsky: It seems quite probable that a year of political paralysis and constitutional crisis would have been averted altogether if, at several crucial junctures in their respective lives, either the fat boy from Hope or the zaftig princess from Beverly Hills had simply been allowed to eat what they wanted to eat, without the accompanying message that their mutual propensity for a certain mild plumpness would mark them as outsiders, if not actual pariahs. Yet in a culture in which "fat" people *are* the new pariahs, that option was never available to them. Nor was it available to the first lady who took away the president's French chef, understanding as she did the limits of what can be tolerated in American political life today. And it is not available to the tens of millions of Americans who struggle every day with the same anxieties and obsessions that helped shape the lives and destinies of the players who found themselves at the center of this strange and compelling political drama: a drama that, ultimately, was perhaps more about fat than it was about anything else.

16

Feminist Accused of
Unsightly Weight Gain

A S THE PREVIOUS CHAPTER ATTESTS, this book was born of an investigation into the Clinton-Lewinsky scandal. The deeper I delved into that topic, the more I discovered the extent to which anxieties about food, fat, weight, and body image seemed to play major roles in the lives and actions of the principal actors in that drama.

I began to become especially intrigued by the question of weight in America when I encountered some striking examples of the effects of our national obsession at the center of my own field. In the summer and fall of 1998, I found myself playing the part of an expert commentator on a number of television talk shows, commenting on aspects of the Clinton-Lewinsky affair. I had just published my book *Jurismania: The Madness of American Law*, and the publisher thought becoming a media commentator on this most spectacular of the Clinton sex-and-politics scandals would be a good way of drumming up publicity. The thesis of the book was that the American legal system was in many ways out of control; and naturally I had no trouble adapting this idea to the goings-on of that overwrought year.

Over the next few months I appeared a number of times on the *Jim Lehrer NewsHour*, *Hardball with Chris Matthews*, CNN, and the like. In the course of these adventures, I got to know something about the world of political punditry, especially as it manifests itself on what has been called "infotainment television." I also started watching these programs regularly. As an occasional guest I was particularly interested in the performances of the "regulars"—the commentators who often appeared several times per week. And, partly for personal reasons, I was especially struck by the dynamic between two women who seemed to be paired up against each other night after night.

Ann Coulter had been a law school classmate of mine. The Lewinsky affair soon propelled her to the position of alpha female among a bevy of telegenic right-wing commentators: a group of conventionally attractive young women television critics had dubbed the "pundettes." Coulter, whose flowing blonde locks seem to have become much blonder in the decade since law school, is very tall, very thin (she has been quoted in the press discussing her size 0 jeans), and very strident. Unlike most attorneys who appear on these sorts of programs, her hatred for the opposition (in this case Bill Clinton and his supporters) seemed quite genuine and indeed visceral.

Night after night, she would pop up on *Rivera Live* or *Hardball*, tossing her platinum mane in a coquettish wave before the camera's hungry lens, and spitting verbal venom toward the president and his defenders. Whether Coulter is actually attractive is a matter of opinion, but there is no doubt that her appeal to television producers was driven by the fact that her appearance conformed to various aspects of the cultural ideal. Coulter's professional credentials for her role were almost as slender as her figure: She had quit her job as a junior lawyer for a big New York firm to come to Washington, and at the time she didn't seem to have any regular employment beyond appearing on political talk shows (where she was identified rather vaguely as a "constitutional attorney").

To be blunt, what Coulter had to sell to television producers was that she was a conventionally attractive (i.e., extraordinarily thin) young woman with a law degree, some strong opinions, and a willingness to express them in no uncertain terms. These credentials were enough to make her a talk show television star: a role she subsequently parlayed into the authorship of a pair of best-selling books and a syndicated opinion column. In the words of another pundette, Heather Nauert (and to be fair, Nauert sometimes makes Coulter sound like Hannah Arendt), "it's more interesting to see a young person talking about issues than a big old fat white guy."

The structure of political talk shows more or less requires that someone such as Coulter be paired up against an appropriate opponent. Throughout the summer and fall of 1998, Coulter's attacks on Clinton were most often parried by Susan Estrich. Unlike Coulter, Estrich possessed a dazzling array of academic, professional, and political credentials: In the mid-1970s she had become the first woman ever elected president of the *Harvard Law Review*, meaning that she had secured the most prestigious student position available at the nation's top law school. She had then gone on to become one of the first women to join the Harvard Law School faculty, where she wrote a path-breaking book on rape in America, based in part on her own experiences as a victim of that crime. Subsequently, she became the first woman to manage a major presidential campaign (that of Michael Dukakis).

In the years since, she had moved to the University of Southern California Law School, and written a book on criminal procedure entitled *Getting Away with Murder*. At the height of the Lewinsky scandal this book was co-reviewed with *Jurismania* in the *Los Angeles Times*; and watching Coulter and Estrich perform night after night upon the same stage on which I occasionally appeared, I found myself experiencing a certain odd sense of connection with both my former classmate and present colleague. But more than that, I was fascinated by the contrasts and the similarities between these two women—between the pundette and the professor, each of whom clearly relished the role she had been assigned to play.

My fascination only grew when I discovered that Susan Estrich had just written a diet book, of all things. And, when I actually read *Making the Case for Yourself: A Diet Book for Smart Women*, I began to understand the extent to which, as the feminist slogan puts it, the personal truly is political. Consider the following passage from Professor Estrich's diet book—a passage that all but refers to Coulter by name:

> Sometimes I find myself in these strange partnerships of left and right on television against women of really great beauty, who clearly spend much more time on their hair in preparation for these encounters than I did on mine for dinner with the president. Are we now choosing female pundits for beauty, not for experience, insight and acumen? Where are all my old friends from [political campaigns], all the women who are still eating five meals a day as they drag themselves across the country? How come I'm never paired with good-looking men?

These are excellent questions. Coming as they do from someone who has been considered a notable figure in the feminist movement, one might expect they would lead to answers that would reject the various premises that fuel the public culture that has given birth to, among other things, pundettes. But one would be wrong.

Making the Case for Yourself is a profoundly antifeminist book, under even the loosest definition of what might be considered feminism. Considering the identity of its author, its contents should have caused a scandal. Instead it went on to become one of the best-selling diet books of the year, while provoking barely a ripple of reaction among those who should have been outraged by its message. It is a text that deserves close attention, if only to illustrate the extent to which the culture of thinness has overwhelmed even people who ought to be leading the protest against that culture's oppressive grip.

The book begins with a claim that did draw some notice, so egregiously did it violate the norms of feminist opinion. After supplying her readers with an appropriately long list of her professional accomplishments, Estrich makes the following confession: "Nothing that I do now or have done in the past . . . has made me prouder, happier, or more fulfilled than losing weight and getting in shape." On one level—apparently, given the rest of the book, a subconscious one—this statement must be read as a confession, if only because it is so appalling. That someone who is among the half dozen most distinguished women lawyers of her generation should openly admit to taking more pride in moving from a size 12 to a size 6 ("sometimes a 4") dress than in any of her professional accomplishments is tantamount to an admission that she has simply surrendered to the cultural judgment that, in terms of her value as a person, nothing a woman does can ever be as important as her appearance.

Now in a way (a rather sick way) there is something admirable about this confession. For one thing, there can be no doubt that it is true, in the sense that it reflects the author's genuine beliefs. Furthermore, it's a confession that many other women in positions comparable to Estrich's would also make, if they were to choose to be as candid about such a sensitive subject. Indeed, when I asked for her reaction to Estrich's statement, an equally accomplished law professor (not the professor quoted to similar effect in Chapter 14) told me, "Truthfully, lots of us who struggle to stay thin have felt that way, at least some of the time. The difference is we would be ashamed to admit it."

Far from being consciously ashamed of finding herself in the grip of this attitude, Estrich revels in it. Over and over again, she affirms that she only feels good about herself when she "looks good," and she only "looks good" when she fits into a size 6—or on a good day, size 4—(the average American woman wears a size 12 to 14): "I don't want to convince you that looking good [by this she means being thin] is a slightly foolish obsession that properly centered, successful women can ill afford. I want to convince you of just the opposite." And she proceeds to put her considerable forensic talents to work to do just that.

Making the Case for Yourself features three interrelated narratives: an autobiography describing twenty-five years of failed diets followed by a final redemption from the purgatory of the size 12 dress; a series of arguments regarding why attaining slimness should be a major life goal for otherwise successful professional women; and a plan of action designed to enable the reader to achieve a life-transforming loss of weight. It is, in other words, a typical and indeed clichéd representative of its genre. What makes this particular collection of clichés interesting is the social identity of its author.

Estrich describes growing up in a middle-class Jewish milieu that had more than a little in common with that satirized by novelists such as Philip Roth ("My mother deals with life by worrying . . . if she leaves a message that doesn't begin with, 'Everything's all right,' I know that it isn't"). What Estrich's mother mostly worried about, it seems, was her daughters' weight:

> My mother considered it her job to watch everything we ate, to make sure we wouldn't get fat. It worked, sort of. I grew up always believing I was on the fat side, never confident that I looked just fine. Now I look at old pictures, and I don't get it. I look thin.

It's difficult for anyone who has ever looked critically at the diet culture to read such passages (and there are many in this book) without becoming exasperated. To be blunt, how can someone with an IQ that's no doubt four or so standard deviations to the right side of the mean manage to produce such a painfully naive interpretation of the evidence? Not once on any of the book's two-hundred-odd pages is there any hint that it has occurred to Estrich that her "weight problem" might be a problem of self-image rather than of physiology.

Anyway, Estrich relates that she first got "fat" when she went off to college at Wellesley, a very elite, very WASP college where she gained weight, finished her freshman year at 140 pounds, and then proceeded to spend the next three years spending her mother's money by bouncing between diet doctors and Weight Watchers, in a desperate attempt to avoid being the fat Jewish girl among the *shikse* princesses. ("My mother refused to send me back to college fat . . . We didn't have a lot of money, but this was important to us.") Thus began the all-too-familiar saga of the yo-yo dieter, as the future Harvard professor fluctuated between a few pounds above her "ideal" weight (at no point in the book does she reveal what this mysterious figure is supposed to be) and the dreaded 140 pounds.

When as an undergraduate she weighed 140 pounds, Estrich considered herself a "blob"—and she still employs much the same judgment today. This refusal to adjust for context is typical of lifetime dieters, who cling to the irrational belief—a belief reinforced by the propaganda of the weight loss industry—that there is no reason why a middle-aged mother ought to weigh more than she did when she was a childless college student a quarter century earlier. Interestingly, Estrich never discloses how tall she is: For her the number on the scale seems to be some sort of Platonic figure, detached from any concession to the fact that any evaluation of weight is largely meaningless if it doesn't account for height.

As we shall see, it's no coincidence that Estrich never mentions body mass index, or any other scientific—or rather, pseudoscientific—basis for her claims that she was, objectively speaking, "fat." Instead, she goes on to describe her years at Harvard Law School, which she entered at what she considered a barely acceptable weight (unstated, but obviously below 140), and left "fat," after being unable to combine strict dieting with the eighty-hour workweeks required of the president of the *Harvard Law Review*. She was not merely the first woman in that position: She was the only woman in her class on the *Review,* and she relates that other women law students "saw it as their responsibility to keep me going, to buck me up when a third-year student called me an 'ambitious chick' and to bring me brownies, sandwiches, lasagne, and other taste treats."

Then it was off to a top law firm, a Supreme Court clerkship, a position on the Harvard faculty, and more yo-yo dieting. In the fall of 1987 she was picked to head Michael Dukakis's presidential campaign ("I looked pretty good on the day Governor Dukakis announced my appointment, which would turn out to be my thinnest moment of the next five years"). The inevitable chaos of a presidential campaign made it impossible for her to diet strictly, and naturally she gained weight. A few months later she discovered she was pregnant with her first child.

Estrich goes on to relate that she "gained 40 pounds during my first pregnancy, lost 30, and then gained 40-plus during my second. You see how the math works . . . I had plateaued at fat." It was then, a few months after the birth of her second child, that she went on a diet and stayed on it for at least three years, reducing her weight to 130 pounds, and inspiring her to share the secrets of her success in book form.

Several features of Estrich's life as a dieter are worth noting. First, like the majority of people who try to lose weight, Estrich was never actually fat by any sane definition of that term. Estrich appears to be of average height, which means that when she was a self-described 140-pound "blob" her BMI was probably within the recommended range of 18.5 to 24.9 promulgated by the scare-mongering bureaucrats who prosecute the war on fat. Indeed, the highest non-pregnant weight she ever reached in her life—apparently around 160 pounds—was barely enough to qualify her as marginally overweight, even by the absurdly restrictive and scientifically baseless standards of the BMI tables; and she was certainly never anywhere near a weight that a rational medical analysis would begin to consider problematic in its own right. Estrich was "fat," in other words, in only two closely related places: in her own mind, and in the context of a culture (contemporary America in general, and Southern California in particular) that has enshrined a medically dangerous degree of thinness as the feminine ideal.

Second, Estrich's pattern of dieting over a twenty-five-year period— losing weight and then gaining it back, plus a bit more, over and over again—is the long-term pattern followed by most dieters. That she characterizes a three-year period of lower weight following on the heels of the previous quarter century of yo-yo dieting as a story of failure followed by success is understandable as a matter of personal psychology but unwarranted from the perspective of social analysis. As of the date of her book's publication Estrich had spent more than 90% of her adult life failing to diet successfully, and less than 10% of that time maintaining a relatively long-term lower weight. This percentage happens to mirror roughly the percentage of dieters who manage to successfully maintain long-term weight loss. In other words, if we think of Susan Estrich not as a single individual but as a succession of dieters moving in one body through time, her story merely reflects that of dieters in general—a fact obscured by the detail that she wrote her book at the precise moment when her narrative lent itself to reinterpretation as a story of long-term failure followed at long last by "permanent" success.

Third, remarkably for a self-identified feminist, Estrich never notes the obvious political implications of the common theme that links the times in her life when she was least able to diet and therefore gained the most weight: when she was president of the *Harvard Law Review*, and when she ran the Dukakis campaign. Her book makes clear that these are her proudest professional accomplishments (she also makes clear that the proudest moments of her personal life involved giving birth to and raising her children, which not coincidentally happens to be the other stage of her life during which she gained the most weight). "I look at my dieting history," she notes, "and the moral is pretty clear. The harder I worked, the fatter I got." Someone who was less in the grip of the dieting culture would be able to draw a more explicit moral: The more Estrich worked like a high-powered professional man, the less time and energy she had available to dedicate to attempts to force her body to conform to an arbitrary and oppressive cultural ideal.

Estrich is quite clear about one aspect of dieting: If you want to lose weight it has to be a full-time job. "On a scale of 1 to 10," she asks her readers, "how important is it for you to lose weight and get in shape?" (The book contains no hint that these two goals might not be identical.) "Don't think. Give me a number. If it's lower than 9 (we'll reserve 10 for your family's good health, solvency and world peace), you're not ready and you're going to fail." Estrich tells readers that among other things they need to "write a memo to the file" every night, evaluating what they ate that day, why, how they felt when they ate it, and so on. She brushes aside potential objections that her dieting strategies are quite time consuming ("this is a 9 on a 1 to 10 scale; we've already had this conversation"). And she is correct about this: A person who wants to maintain a body weight 10 or 20 or 30 pounds below what she would maintain if she engaged in normal eating—that is, eating food that she likes when she's hungry, and stopping when she's full—will only be able to do so by maintaining the sort of hyper-vigilance that Estrich identifies as the key to successful dieting. (Over and over again, the book emphasizes to mothers who work for income that they must accept the necessity of performing three full-time jobs: employee, mother, and dieter.)

In other words, unlike diet book authors who promise painless weight loss, Estrich doesn't sugarcoat the fact that dieting is hard work, and work that has to be done on a daily—if not hourly—basis for the rest of the successful dieter's life. Indeed, she admits that her own sense of accomplishment springs from the massive exercise of willpower she must put forth every day:

> I can't eat whatever I want. If I do, I will get fat. I wish that weren't true . . . I think fudge tastes great. I love rich chocolate, bagels and cream cheese, any kind of bread . . . I like wine, peanuts and pizza . . . I don't want to think about this any more . . . If someone told me tomorrow that I could eat anything I wanted and be slim and healthy, I would not eat oatmeal with skim milk for breakfast. Not even close. Waffles with syrup and butter one day, an apple pancake the next. I would not eat steamed vegetables for lunch or grilled chicken for dinner. Who's kidding whom?

This grim confession naturally leads to the question of exactly why the reader ought to rank undertaking a Herculean effort to achieve and maintain an otherwise unattainable weight the fourth most important thing in the world, right behind her family's health, avoiding poverty and, as the beauty pageant contestants remind us every year, "world peace." What could possibly justify dedicating a large part of one's life to avoiding such fundamental pleasures as bread, chocolate, and wine?

Estrich has two basic answers to this question: protecting your health and salvaging your self-esteem. Over and over again, *Making the Case for Yourself* hammers home the message that dieting is all about making sure you live long enough to see your children grow up. According to Estrich, the mother who is 20 or 30 pounds "overweight" and refuses to diet is as irresponsible as a heroin addict, and for the same reason: because her self-indulgence threatens to leave her children orphaned at an early age. Here's the advice she gives readers faced with the hypothetical temptation of a croissant: "If everybody else at the table were shooting heroin, would you? If they were committing slow suicide, would you? . . . Eating it is suicidal. Which is worse, wasting a croissant, or using it to speed up your death, and make your hips fat?"

To the charge that this kind of rhetoric will fill people with guilt, Estrich is only too eager to plead guilty. Indeed, she presents guilt as the second item (behind vanity) in her list of reasons to lose weight: "Guilt . . ." As in, "You have two young children, how can you not take care of yourself? How can you increase the chance that you won't be here when they need you?" Like some sort of parody of a Jewish mother, she keeps coming back to this theme: "Would you like to watch your children grow up or not? Are you going to do everything you can to live a longer, healthier life, or a shorter one in a wheelchair? Have you thrown away that croissant yet?"

All of this, of course, is absurd. There is not a shred of scientific evidence that a 160-pound woman of average height who is physically active and eats a reasonably balanced diet will have worse long-term health prospects than women of similar height who weigh 30 pounds less, and who also have healthy lifestyles. Indeed, the heavier woman will have far *better* health, on average, than the thinner women, if the latter are sedentary. And while *Making the Case for Yourself* talks a good deal about exercise, it always does so in the context of emphasizing how crucial exercise is to losing weight. Nothing in Estrich's book indicates she is aware that the health benefits of exercise appear to be almost completely independent of whether it results in any weight loss.

Estrich's attitude toward exercise is typical of people who work out primarily to lose weight: She hates it. In a nice metaphor for a number of things, she managed to bribe herself to ride a stationary bike for forty-five minutes a day by indulging in simultaneous fantasies of consumption and reduction: "I didn't exercise; I shopped. I sat on my bike and read catalogues. I fantasized about the clothes I was going to wear when I was thin . . . I rode my bike rather than doing my half of the taxes; there's always something even less appealing than exercise." It's unnecessary to point out that almost all people who engage in strenuous physical activity on such a basis will be unable to maintain a commitment to it, no matter how many lectures about "slow suicide" they may hear from those prosecuting the case against fat.

One of the most striking aspects of *Making the Case for Yourself* is its failure to cite any support for its histrionic health warnings. Of course one doesn't expect to find solid arguments for medical assertions in the typical diet book, but when the book in question has been authored by the Charles Kingsley Professor of Law and Political Science at a major research university, one would think readers have a right to expect something more. Instead, Estrich merely asserts that everyone knows fat kills: "You don't need the doctor to tell you to lose weight. Presumably, you know you should. You don't even need him to explain the risks. You probably know them, and can easily research them." However easy this research may be to do, it's clear that Estrich either hasn't done it herself, or has chosen to misrepresent what that research reveals about the connections between weight and health. For example, one would never guess from reading Estrich's book that eight million Americans suffer from eating disorders, or that the health effects of precisely the sort of yo-yo dieting she has spent almost all of her adult life engaging in are far worse than all but the most extreme levels of obesity. (The words "anorexia" and "bulimia" do not appear in her text, and the phrase "eating disorder" is used only once, in the context of discussing binge eating.)

Yet as inaccurate as *Making the Case for Yourself* is as a source for advice on health and fitness, the noxious character of this part of the book pales in comparison to Estrich's arguments regarding self-esteem. For ultimately, Estrich's argument is directed more toward her readers' emotional—rather than physical—well-being. And it is this part of the narrative that crosses the line that separates the badly misinformed from the genuinely outrageous. Losing weight, Estrich emphasizes, is not merely or even primarily about "saving your life." It is about saving "your marriage, your sense of self-esteem." And just in case the reader is failing to make the connection between these topics, the text includes such useful nuggets of information as, "Did you know that most married men who have affairs do so within a year of the birth of their second child?" It has come to this: The cult of dieting has become so all-encompassing that one of the leading feminist legal scholars of her generation is now giving out advice on how to lose 20 pounds in order to hold your man, and no one even blinks.

It gets worse. Consider Estrich's tips on how to charm rich and powerful men at formal dinners, using methods that have the added bonus of not allowing courtesans who are genuinely committed to their craft any time to actually eat:

> Pamela Harriman, the wife and lover of many of the greatest, richest, most powerful men of her century, was widely regarded as one of the sexiest women of our times . . . Harriman always looked good, and she got slimmer as she got older, which is the way you have to do it. But what's always struck me is that every man who has ever sat next to her at dinner tells exactly the same drippy story. "I know it sounds trite," they would say, in an apt description of how it sounded. "But when she was sitting next to you, you thought you were the most attractive, interesting, intelligent, sexy man in the room." It was how she made men feel about themselves that they always remembered . . . She was charming, and part of her charm was that she made these guys feel like they were ten feet tall, or long. Figuring out how to make a person interesting—to themselves, and to you—is a much bigger challenge than letting them bore you both . . . Believe me it leaves you no time to eat.

As horrifying as all this is, a passage such as this displays, I suppose, a certain commendable honesty. At least Estrich admits that, in the context of what Naomi Wolf has termed the cult of dieting, "maintaining good self-esteem" is more or less a synonym for doing whatever is necessary to acquire and hold onto a suitably status-enhancing man. Nevertheless, whatever the virtues of this sort of candor might be, they don't begin to compensate for the frightening fact that a woman who is considered something of an icon of a certain brand of feminism feels emboldened to publish things that might strike the editors of *Cosmopolitan* as being a touch retrograde—and when she does, it elicits barely a peep of protest.

The most disturbing part of Estrich's argument is that at the same time her own life provides an excellent illustration of why almost all dieters fail, and why people who diet end up, on average, weighing

more than people of similar initial weight who don't, she remains blind
to the perverse paradox she is describing. Diets fail for many reasons,
but perhaps the single most important is that succeeding at any difficult long-term project requires feeling good about those aspects of
oneself such a project engages. No novel worth reading was ever written by anyone who didn't believe he was a good novelist. The sick
irony at the heart of the diet culture is captured in Estrich's statement
that "the easiest way to diet, and maybe the only way, is to do it as part
of a larger, positive, immediately rewarding effort to reconnect with
your body in a beneficial way." Yet Estrich remains oblivious to the
point that, for the vast majority of people, reconnecting with their bodies in a beneficial way requires accepting the simple truth that *there
is actually nothing wrong with their bodies in the first place.* In other
words, as generations of ex-dieters have discovered, for most people
"the only way" to deal with their weight successfully is not to diet
at all.

Estrich seems to be on the verge of something like this insight
when she notes, "Every single survey of men and every self-help article
for women comes down to the same point on sexiness. You are what
you think you are. Sexy women are women who think they're sexy.
They are women who like their bodies. If you think you're sexy, you
are." But then it all goes wrong: "A sexy woman is a woman who
likes her body so of course she takes care of it which makes her lose
weight which makes her like her body even more which makes her
even sexier which makes her exercise more which makes her lose
more weight . . ." A more precise description of the theoretical pretzel
logic behind the practice of anorexia and bulimia would be difficult
to formulate.

Even within the context of the doublethink so characteristic of the
diet culture, the level of cognitive dissonance at the center of Estrich's
arguments is breathtaking. Again, at the same time that she recognizes
such truths as that there isn't "a single woman alive who doesn't do
better, personally and professionally, when she feels *great* about herself," and that the key to a fulfilling life is to choose "to be your best, to
be happy with yourself, to be fit and strong and self-confident for
however long you are blessed to be here" she steadfastly refuses to acknowledge the empirically undeniable fact that, for almost all people—
indeed, for Susan Estrich herself, until a couple of years before she wrote

this book—feeling great about themselves and being fit and strong and self-confident precludes the whole idea of dieting, which at its core is all about weakness and self-loathing and endless dissatisfaction.

Estrich doesn't see things this way. She doesn't deny that trying and failing to lose weight is often psychologically devastating to those who, like her, have dedicated much of their lives to going on and falling off an endless series of diets. Her solution to this problem is never go off your diet: "We've all got problems . . . but being fat and unhealthy and hating yourself are three additional problems that you could live without." Of course this line of reasoning is simply an insult to both the author's and the reader's intelligence, and in a number of ways. Let us count some of them.

The notion that thinness equals fitness, and fat equals ill health, is demonstrably false. Now it's true that most Americans believe this (I believed it when I began to research this book). On the other hand, an academic of all people has no excuse for not actually examining the evidence before writing a book that advises its readers about the very health issues in regard to which Estrich appears to have maintained an almost complete ignorance.

Estrich is a professor of law and political science. She is also a national figure in Democratic Party politics. Given this, it's reasonable to assume that, when faced with a social practice that for more than a century has consistently left the vast majority of those who engage in it worse off than they were prior to the attempt, her reaction is normally something other than to advise people to keep trying until they get it right. Would she, for example, advocate eliminating Social Security on the grounds that there has never been any need for such a program, given that sufficiently self-disciplined people have always been able to save enough money for retirement? That is the sort of claim one might expect from, say, a not terribly bright libertarian, rather than from anyone blessed with a modicum of insight regarding the nature of human beings. Yet this is precisely her advice to failing dieters. It never occurs to her to grapple with the obvious question: If this advice is worth giving, why did she herself spend more than twenty years taking it to no avail?

If, as Estrich acknowledges, self-hatred is a product of failure, and failure is a product of the nature of the enterprise, how difficult is it to figure out that the problem isn't the failure of the enterprise, but the enterprise itself? For almost all people who struggle with their weight, dieting results in failure, which produces unhappiness, which leads to compensatory bingeing, which produces more unhappiness, and so on and so forth, until you've produced a nation that features 115 million dieters and 135 million "overweight" people, with most of the people in the former category also belonging to the latter group. Indeed, this neurotic cycle probably plays a larger role in making people fatter than they would otherwise be than any other single cultural factor in America today. Simply put, dieting causes the condition it's supposed to cure. Most people who diet would be happier, healthier, and thinner if they never dieted. This group included Susan Estrich for much of her adult life, and is likely to include her again.

Estrich must find some way of denying all this, of course. Her preferred strategy for denying the hard truths about dieting is, well, denial:

> Why do we search for miracle cures when Western medicine can tell you how to lose weight? . . . It is perverse. There is no other word for it. We want to lose weight, we know how to lose weight, we know it's important to lose weight, we beat ourselves up if we don't lose weight, we have the power to lose weight, we spend money we don't have to lose weight, and we still fail.

And why is that? According to Estrich, it's because "we" are suffering from a contemptible combination of laziness and neurosis:

> You are not fat because you have a hard life. You are not fat because you have a slow metabolism. You are not fat because you are poor, harried, hurt, lonely, overworked, stressed out, depressed, or disabled. You may have been victimized, but you're not doomed to be a victim. You are fat because you don't eat right, and don't exercise enough, for you.

All of this assumes the existence of imaginary human beings, rather than the ones who actually inhabit the United States at the beginning of the twenty-first century. If there is one thing that is not in doubt about "Western medicine," it is that it cannot tell people how to successfully lose weight. And if there is one thing that is not in doubt about contemporary Americans is that tens of millions of them are sincerely desperate to achieve a culturally approved weight, and they will try almost anything, including many things that endanger their health, in the depths of their desperation to achieve that perverse and ultimately self-destructive goal.

I dislike being forced to criticize a colleague so bluntly. But I must admit that there is a part of me—the part that watches my beautiful nine-year-old daughter doing her karate kata, or modeling her new outfit in front of a full-length mirror, her physical self-esteem still intact for a few more precious months or years—that wants to grab Susan Estrich by the metaphorical lapels of her size 6 suit, and scream, *How is it possible for a person of your intelligence to be so blind? Surely there must be some level of consciousness at which you have some inkling of just how perverse, wrongheaded, and ultimately destructive the things you are saying actually are.*

That, however, would not be very constructive. I do wish there was some way to take part in a conversation that would explore why people such as Estrich believe they have found the key to weight loss, when the advice she gives on the matter is no different than that which she herself was unable to follow, and that left her struggling with the misery of the diet treadmill for so many years.

Anyway, how exactly is "Susan's Miracle Diet" (I'm not making that title up) supposed to work its miraculous transformation, when almost all diets fail? Given that it is the work of a law professor, it should come as no surprise that the actual diet plan presented by *Making the Case for Yourself* is a nice example of naive rationalism run amok—a kind of Restatement of Sacher Torts. The author's interpretation of her recent sustained weight loss is that it was a product of finally outsmarting the demons of weight gain with an appropriately harsh regimen of bright line rules: "Someone asked me how I'd lost all that weight. 'The same way she does everything else [Estrich quotes a friend as saying]. She used her brain.' " In other words, Estrich understands her previous twenty-five years of recurrent dietary disaster as the product of an intellectual failure. This of course is completely implausible; and in fact the autobiographical section of the book portrays the author spending decades on the kind of comprehensive dieting research project that hyperintellectual, pragmatically minded persons such as Estrich specialize in undertaking, as she searched constantly for the weight loss formula that would actually "work."

What finally worked for Estrich, at least temporarily, was nothing new, but rather a collection of the most basic tenets of dieting: Come up with strict rules regarding what you can and can't eat in advance, and stick to them no matter what. Eat your vegetables. Don't eat standing up in the kitchen or late at night. Keep a food journal. Exercise regularly. Most important of all, avoid "bad" foods. This doesn't just mean doughnuts either. In order to achieve and maintain a desirable weight, Estrich advises her readers to "always" eat fruits and vegetables, to "sometimes" eat chicken, fish, egg whites, and non-dairy fat, to "rarely" eat potatoes, bread (!), pasta (!!), rice, bagels and oil, and to "never" eat anything else. Consider what "anything else" includes, and take into account that, for people who want to stay 20 pounds below their natural weight, dieting in this fashion is pretty much a life sentence. Is it any wonder that almost all diets fail?

Estrich has convinced herself that all this adds up to some sort of new approach, at least for her, but in fact her own narrative reveals the extent to which she had tried to do all of these things in the past, but had been unable to stick with it. At last, in her early forties, she suddenly found herself able to deny herself all sorts of foods that she had never been able to deny herself before, even though they made her "fat" (i.e., 20 pounds over an arbitrary cultural ideal).

Why was she finally able to do this, at least for a few years, after a quarter century of failure? "Western medicine" still has no idea why some people manage to stick to diets for years or even decades, while most people can't. Needless to say Estrich has no idea either, but lifetime dieters tend to be rationalists, and rationalists tend to find the answers they need, even when those answers are obviously being manufactured out of the thinnest air. Predictably, Estrich ascribes her success to the same qualities that have served her so well in her career: a talent for breaking down problems analytically, a capacity for hard work, considerable reserves of sheer willpower, and so on. The question she neither answers nor asks is, why did these talents, which were so clearly part of her makeup during the two-plus decades when she engaged in yo-yo dieting, suddenly prove adequate to the task after having failed her so many times before? *Making the Case for Yourself* does not and cannot answer that most basic of all the mysteries that beset the cult of dieting.

The saddest aspect of this book is implicit in the quotation with which I began: a passage from the book's last page, in which Estrich appears to be revealing the deepest motivations behind this strange and disturbing text. When the author concludes with the observation that "sometimes I find myself in these strange partnerships of left and right on television against women of really great beauty," we can be fairly sure she is getting close to the heart of the matter. I've said some harsh things about Susan Estrich in this chapter, all of which were deserved. Nevertheless, a part of me recognizes that, as a woman colleague put it, "Susan is also a victim" of the malignant cultural forces that *Making the Case for Yourself* unfortunately reflects and extends. Somewhere underneath the presumption and arrogance and naiveté of the high-status lawyer giving advice regarding things she doesn't understand, there is no doubt still some psychic echo of the girl who agonized about fitting in with the popular crowd, or getting a date to the prom, or being callously dumped by someone whom she suspected would have behaved differently if she looked more like the Ann Coulters of this world.

Perhaps the greatest irony underlying such suspicions is this: Ann Coulter is not a woman of really great beauty. Ann Coulter is tall and extremely thin and has very long blonde hair. That's it. That doesn't add up to beauty. Mostly, Coulter is beautiful in the eyes of people who equate female beauty with little more than being a tall thin blonde woman. Furthermore, a lot of men actually prefer the 20 pounds Estrich has spent her life trying to lose. (Studies indicate that women tend to underestimate what the typical man considers the most desirable body type for women by about 20 pounds.) Coulter has even complained recently that she can't get a date from among all the eligible men in Washington, D.C. This is not, in fact, particularly surprising. Because ultimately, as shallow and superficial as men can be about these sorts of things (and that's saying something), most of us are not *that* shallow.

When I first read *Making the Case for Yourself*, I was appalled and angered. For one thing, the thought that my daughter is growing up in a culture that leads a woman who was once a prominent feminist scholar to write such a book is extremely disturbing. My anger subsided somewhat when I considered this passage: "Looking at my baby daughter, and three years later my baby son, I understood the elemental power of love, how people could be moved to kill; I would kill anyone who touched them." Those are genuine words, written by a loving parent, struggling despite everything to do her best by those who most depend on her.

What should appall and anger us is not so much Estrich's book, but rather the culture that made it possible. That a woman of such brilliance and accomplishment should waste years of her life agonizing over something as trivial as her inability to lose 20 pounds is an indictment of a society, not an individual. Even so, individuals still have it within their power to undertake potentially heroic acts of resistance. The greatest gift Susan Estrich could give her daughter is the same one each of us can give our own children. And that is to reject the poisonous lie at the heart of the obesity myth: that learning to hate the body you were born with is the key to health, happiness, and a life worth living.

17

Anorexia Nervosa and the
Spirit of Capitalism

THE AMERICAN WEIGHT LOSS INDUSTRY is a fifty-billion-dollar-per-year con game, which for many decades has provided its customers with totally ineffective cures for an imaginary disease. Such an unusual social and economic situation raises a number of interesting questions. How can an industry whose products have a failure rate of around 95%, and that usually leave those who buy them quite a bit worse off, continue to prosper? How does one explain the almost unchallenged power of so many cultural myths about fat, when it rapidly becomes clear to any disinterested person who bothers to study the issue that those myths are based on a combination of the worst sort of junk science, and the most invidious forms of social discrimination? In other words, what is it about fat in America that makes the subject largely impervious to rational discussion and debate?

The obesity myth is rooted in a combination of bad science, psychological biases, and, most decisively, powerful ideological commitments—commitments that are all the more powerful because they are largely unconscious. Ultimately, the ideology that generates so much fear and loathing of fat drives everything else that makes up the war against it: the poorly designed research, the irrational government policies, the shoddy journalism that accepts that research and those policies at face value, and most of all the unwillingness of otherwise skeptical Americans to consider the possibility that the supposed facts they are fed by the weight loss industry, either directly or through their mouthpieces in the government and the media, might be little more than a mixture of gross exaggerations and outright lies.

Fat Science

The study of obesity as a pathological medical condition is a field of research that was founded on the basis of a pair of related hypotheses: that there is a usefully predictable relationship between increasing body mass and decreasing overall health, and that therefore medical science should strive to find ways to make fat people healthier, by helping them become thinner. The weight of more than a half century of research has demolished these assumptions.

Subject to exceptions for extreme cases, even the crude statistical studies that long dominated, and to a great extent still dominate, the field—those that failed to take into account such crucial factors as sedentary lifestyle and the harmful effects of dieting—by and large failed to establish any sort of reliable link between being overweight and having poorer than average health. Indeed, more sophisticated studies have since established that, when such variables are taken into account, fat simply drops out of the equation as a meaningful predictor of health and mortality.

In particular, scientists have by now compiled a mountain of evidence, based on data collected from decades-long studies of tens of thousands of subjects, that fat active people are far healthier than thin sedentary individuals, and that they are in general just as healthy as thin active persons. Given this evidence, it has become clear that, contrary to the founding assumptions of obesity research, there is no necessary contradiction between fatness and fitness, and that slenderness in and of itself has no particular health value. (Just as there is no reason that fatness precludes fitness, there is no reason to believe that slenderness necessarily indicates fitness, either.)

Furthermore, an equally compelling body of evidence indicates that attempts to lose weight do have, on average, a predictable effect on health: a very bad one. For example (one of many), a Swedish study of persons who had been placed on very low-calorie diets—the sort of diet Monica Lewinsky's mother tried to put her on when she was sixteen—found a mortality rate of fifty-nine sudden deaths per one hundred thousand people: forty times the rate of such deaths in the general population. The reaction of mainstream obesity researchers to such data has been particularly illuminating. Perhaps my favorite single example of how much of the work in this field is an embarrassment to the word "science" is provided by an experiment conducted by the Veterans Administration in the 1960s. In this study, almost two hundred very fat young men were placed on radically restrictive diets. Before they entered the study, none of the men had any serious health problems (of course, according to the axioms of mainstream obesity research, all of them were automatically assumed to have a serious health problem, i.e., they were fat). While on the diets the men lost an average of about 75 pounds; typically, almost all of them eventually regained the weight they had lost, plus a little more.

In the years immediately following their participation in the study, these young men suffered a mortality rate that was up to *thirteen times* higher than that of equally heavy men who had not been put on any sort of diet (fifty died, which is forty-six more deaths than would have been expected among men of similar age over this time period). Again, none of the men who died had entered the study with any known health problems. And what was the reaction to this amazing mortality rate? Were there calls for an investigation of a government experiment that seemed to have killed a significant portion of the healthy young men who took part in it? Hardly. In the years since, this study has been cited more than two hundred times in the obesity research literature as evidence for the proposition that "obesity" is a highly dangerous condition, and that patients suffering from it should therefore accept the risks inherent in potentially dangerous treatments!

It is no doubt in some sense true that, as the philosopher Nietzsche put it, "there are no facts, only interpretations." Nevertheless, as interpretations go, this one is, to put the matter in slightly less exalted epistemological terms, nuts. Another interpretation, one supported by many similar experimental outcomes, is that dieting—and especially radical dieting—kills. As two leading dissenters in the obesity research community (Paul Ernsberger and Paul Haskew) have put it, "the astronomical death rate of crash dieters that regain their lost weight [as in fact almost all do] suggests that the hazards associated with fatness may be mainly related to rapid weight loss and regain of weight, not to obesity itself."

The profound deafness so many obesity researchers manifest toward these sorts of suggestions remains, unfortunately, characteristic of much of the field. Indeed, while the field may have been founded on the basis of honest theoretical mistakes, it is by this point too often marked by an apparent willingness to commit increasingly dishonest ones. It isn't much of an exaggeration to say that the basic research program of mainstream obesity studies requires its participants to make all of the following assumptions:

➤ The association between fatness and various diseases proves that fatness causes those diseases.

➤ By contrast, the association between thinness and the equally impressive list of diseases with which thinness is associated is random.

➤ Fat people who become thin acquire the same health characteristics as people who were thin in the first place.

➤ The health risks of attempting to lose weight are justified by the gains to health that losing weight supposedly produces, even when one discounts these supposed benefits by the probability of losing weight successfully.

➤ If fat people were physically active and ate a healthy diet they wouldn't be fat.

It also isn't much of an exaggeration to say that, at the beginning of the twenty-first century, there isn't a shred of evidence for any of these propositions. What, then, accounts for the fact that mainstream obesity studies continue to be funded as if they represented a respectable form of scientific research? Essentially, two factors: economic self-interest and denial.

As for self-interest, it's fairly clear from their off-the-record comments that some putatively orthodox obesity researchers are well aware that much of their field is little more than a scam masquerading as a science. These researchers, however, are also keenly aware that the economics of the field—a field that is almost wholly funded by the weight loss industry—require that the fundamentally flawed premises at the base of most obesity research should never be examined, let alone criticized. Basically, take away the health justification for weight loss and you take away the justification for treating the pursuit of weight loss as a question of medical science. (Medical schools do not grant tenure for research into questions of cosmetology.) And if the claim that fat is a major health risk is allowed to collapse, then the question of fat will be acknowledged to be what it in fact is: an aesthetic question, a social question, and a political question, but not, on the whole, a medical question.

The role denial—in the psychopathological sense of that word— plays in all of this is less crass but more invidious. For one thing, as I have already suggested, the denial some obesity researchers display toward the implications of their own data can be understood as a product of anorexic ideation (i.e., the tendency to interpret the world through an anorexic mental filter). Yet the ideological distortion that marks so much obesity research is too widespread to be explained wholly as a product of individual neurosis. Indeed, having read a good part of their literature, and having interviewed quite a few of them, I can say with some confidence that, for mainstream obesity researchers as a class, the idea that weight in and of itself isn't a significant medical issue is literally *an unthinkable thought.*

Now for the naive rationalist, the idea that there are such things as unthinkable thoughts is disturbing at best, if not downright incomprehensible. Yet consider the social implications of the fact that this same naive rationalist's view of science—a view that imagines researchers going out and gathering raw data in something approaching a purely inductive process, unbiased by prior theoretical assumptions—has by now been effectively discredited by the philosophy of science. As Karl Popper first pointed out more than seventy years ago, the logic of scientific discovery doesn't work that way. Science always proceeds from the initial theoretical intuition to an (always provisional) empirical verification or refutation of that theory, not vice versa.

The implications of this insight for mainstream obesity studies are dire, but clear: Obesity studies were founded on the basis of theoretical intuitions that subsequent empirical investigations have demonstrated were almost completely wrong. Why then have those theories not been discredited? That question assumes the sociology of science is much less complicated than it actually is. Briefly, when a scientific field has managed to organize itself into a durable institutional form— when it has become a separate department within major research universities, when it publishes scholarly journals, when it organizes academic conferences, when it pulls in large grants for undertaking basic research—it can take a very long time for a process of empirical debunking to be reflected by social reality.

For the orthodox obesity researcher, obesity must be a significant health risk, if only because if it were not then it wouldn't make any sense for a field such as obesity studies to exist in anything like its present form. Yet it does exist. And since (again, for a certain type of orthodox rationalist) all forms of knowledge that have managed to institutionalize themselves successfully benefit from an irrebuttable presumption that they aren't organized on the basis of a fundamental theoretical mistake, it follows that the proposition that fat is mostly irrelevant to health is, for this type of thinker, an idea that is literally incredible. By "incredible" I am not using the word, as it is often used, to signify "improbable" or even "undesirable." I mean to say that, for many obesity researchers, their minds will not entertain that idea *at all*. It is ruled out of bounds prior to any interpretation of the evidence.

Indeed, to say it is "ruled out of bounds" makes the process sound more self-conscious than it probably is. For the orthodox obesity researcher, the idea that weight is rarely a significant independent health risk is such self-evident nonsense that it no more needs to be refuted than does the hypothesis that red is bigger than blue, or that C-sharp is heavier than the Pythagorean theorem. As dispiriting as this explanation for the state of mainstream obesity research is, I believe it is the only adequate explanation for how work in this field can continue in the face of so much evidence that its most basic assumptions are deeply mistaken.

Fat Psychology

The corner of Broadway and the Pearl Street Mall in downtown Boulder, Colorado, is one of the epicenters of America's diet and fitness culture. Boulder, a wealthy college town that is also home to many world-class distance runners, triathletes, and rock climbers, is a place where people tend to be concerned to the point of obsession with maintaining a perpetually slim, muscular, and youthful-appearing body. Given the local culture, it's worth noting the businesses that occupy the four street corners at the symbolic center of town. On the east side of Broadway, a Ben & Jerry's ice-cream store and an Abercrombie and

Fitch clothing franchise face each other; on the west side, a Häagen-Dazs and a Banana Republic stare at each other with brown, imperturbable faces.

Inside either of the "super premium" ice-cream stores you can buy a regular cone that is likely to have around 500 calories, or a larger one that will be threatening four caloric figures. As for the clothing stores, they carry almost nothing that the average American, and especially the average American woman, can wear. Having spent quite a few afternoons combing the racks at Banana Republic, the Gap, Ann Taylor, and the like (I suppose by now the local store managers have me pegged for a repressed transvestite), I've discovered that these stores offer merchandise in terms of a sort of standard-distribution bell curve. Beginning with a few size 0 dresses (and we might want to consider the metaphorical, not to mention the metaphysical, implications of offering women's clothing in size 0), the racks tend to fill up with many size 4s and 6s. There are fewer 8s, very few 10s, and maybe a 12 or two. I have yet to find a dress larger than size 12 in any of these stores.

According to industry data, the average American woman wears somewhere between a size 12 and a size 14. Here again we have a social and economic puzzle: a group of retailers whose products fail completely to intersect with the needs of half of the potential market, and the great bulk of whose merchandise can be purchased by about 20% of that market, at most. This situation poses quite a puzzle for traditional models of the relationship between supply and demand. A number of explanations are possible. Perhaps women who shop at relatively expensive places such as Banana Republic and Ann Taylor are much thinner than average (there is good evidence that this is in fact the case, as thinness tends to correlate well with professional and upper-class status). Perhaps higher-end clothing makers find it profitable to shut out a significant portion of the potential market, in return for the indirect economic benefits of having their clothes associated with slenderness. (The recent development of a slew of specialized brands—some of them produced by subsidiaries of the major clothing companies—aimed at the millions of American women wearing sizes 12 and above who have both the desire and the ability to purchase fashionable clothes provides evidence for this explanation as well).

I discovered yet another piece of evidence regarding these issues when I checked out the stock at a Boulder store that specializes in reselling higher-end clothes on consignment. Here, the secondary market for the sorts of dresses available new at Boulder's tonier retailers revealed a selection of dress sizes far closer to the actual needs of the American population. This suggests that there is indeed a significant disjunction between what American women are willing and able to buy in the way of fashionable clothes and the supply structure of the market that makes those clothes available. Which brings us back to the cultural architectonics involved in having two super premium ice-cream stores right next to a couple of shops that offer almost nothing that the average woman who regularly eats super premium ice cream can wear, unless she happens to run marathons or the like.

This sort of commonplace juxtaposition becomes intriguing if we allow ourselves to consider the following idea: In America today, bodies have replaced clothes as the most visible markers of social class. In a culture that combines a high degree of fashion informality with relatively cheap, high-quality clothing, clothes will no longer function as reliable indicators of relative status. On the other hand, a "fit" (misleadingly defined as a slim, toned, and youthful, or at least youthful-appearing) body is much more difficult for the average person to achieve. Acquiring a body that matches this definition of fitness is, for most people, in large part a function of having access to things—health club memberships, personal trainers, plastic surgery, and, most of all, enough energy and leisure time to devote to the pursuit of it—that are far more readily available to professional and upper-class people than they are to the average member of the lower-middle or working classes (let alone to a poor person).

All of which is to say that the average American, and especially the average American woman, runs a daily gauntlet between the siren song of Ben & Jerry's Super Fudge Chunk and the harsh realities of the clothing racks at Banana Republic. She is being bombarded by messages that tempt her to "indulge" in this or that fattening food, while at the same time being told dozens of times a day that fashionable dresses aren't sufficient to display one's social status. After all, people from most ranks of society can now afford fairly fashionable clothes. To be able to afford to make the sacrifices necessary to fit into a size 4, however—that, as Susan Estrich's diet book made so painfully clear, is another matter.

In the America of today, the hardest thing many people ever do is to stay thin. In a nation that supersizes everything, from SUVs to

McDonald's "value" meals, and that eroticizes food to the point where eating a scoop of ice cream becomes a kind of quasi-sexualized transgression, staying thin represents for millions of contemporary Americans a genuine triumph of the will. Imagine how difficult it would be for many of these people to admit that they have spent much of their lives suffering "for nothing"—or worse yet, that the daily and indeed hourly acts of self-denial they have found the psychic strength to perform were not justified by any valid health concerns, but were in fact undertaken in the pursuit of an arbitrary and oppressive cultural ideal.

This, I believe, helps explain the mixed record of almost all mainstream feminist organizations on the issue of fat oppression. Groups such as NOW have done much to point out how media images of extreme thinness help promote the current epidemic of eating disorders among American girls and women, and many individual feminists, such as Naomi Wolf and Susan Bordo, have written devastating critiques of the myriad ways absurdly restrictive body ideals oppress women in general. Yet mainstream feminist groups have focused almost exclusively on the pressures faced by thin, or average weight, or so-called mildly overweight women. Such groups have been almost completely silent about the far greater levels of discrimination so-called obese women in particular face because they are supposedly "too fat"—a silence that radical groups such as Fat Underground have been denouncing since the 1970s.

At bottom, then, the psychological rationalizations that underlie the fear and loathing of fat are, as we saw in the case of Susan Estrich's diet book, crucially linked to the claim that fat kills. Without the psychic and ideological protection provided by that claim, many people—particularly women who identify themselves on at least some level with feminism—would be forced to confront the actual reasons why they have made the sacrifices necessary to conform to the current cultural ideal in regard to weight. And that, in the end, would be a far too painful thing for many of these people to face. That is why much of the most powerful criticism of those ideals has not come from mainstream feminists in size 6 dresses, but from women like Marilyn Wann, Sondra Solovay, Jennifer Portnick, and Carol Wiley, who live every day with the overwhelming prejudice that fat people—not the tens of millions of people who think they "need" to lose 10 or 20 pounds, but *fat* people—face in contemporary America.

These women, who are among the "very vocal minority of super-obese [sic] female activists" that people such as Greg Critser blame for the fattening of America, are genuinely heroic individuals. They are the current cultural equivalent of those professional-class men in business suits who, in the 1950s, would occasionally march in a very small, very orderly picket line, while advocating the outrageous idea that a homosexual person ought to be treated as something other than a disgusting pervert. We can only hope that, one day, the similar sort of courage displayed by fat activists in contemporary America is recognized for what it is: a continuation of the nation's great tradition of producing dissenters who are willing to do battle—at whatever cost to themselves—with the social injustices of their time.

Fat Ideology

Fear and loathing of fat are fueled directly by both bad science and the various forms of denial that interfere with the debunking of the myths this science helps nurture. Nevertheless, these factors by themselves do not explain the depth and intensity of the war on fat. After all, there are many medical research programs whose economic interests would be served by the systematic mischaracterization of the data those programs generate; and there are many other areas of life in which people are given strong incentives not to face up to the reasons why they choose to make the decisions they make. Yet these factors would not normally lead to anything as irrational as our national obsession with "obesity" (a rare case of a comparable outbreak of cultural hysteria is evidenced by the billions of dollars the government spends combating the largely benign practice of smoking marijuana). What is it about fat that makes the distortion surrounding this issue so difficult to combat?

In America today, having a fat body is essentially a fashion faux pas that has been transformed into both a disease and a severe moral failing. Fundamentally, the very idea of fat disgusts the nation's social, economic, and media elites; and disgust is always a morally charged emotion. The emotions fat elicits are fraught with the classic features produced by that which disgusts us: repulsion, fear of contamination, and a morally freighted desire to destroy the thing that disgusts. Thus the basic question that must be answered when attempting to understand the fear of fat in America today is, what are the sources of the profound disgust so many people feel when they confront the thought of a fat body? (Bear in mind that, for tens of millions of Americans today, a "fat" body includes many bodies that would not have been considered fat in almost any other time or place.)

In his famous essay "Protestant Asceticism and the Spirit of Capitalism," the great German sociologist Max Weber put forth an arresting thesis: that there was a critical link between certain Protestant religious doctrines, particularly those espoused by John Calvin and the English Puritans, and the kind of lifestyle best suited for the accumulation of capital through commercial activity. Specifically, Weber argued that the peculiar brand of Christian asceticism advocated by some of the most influential religious leaders of the seventeenth century played a crucial role in the development of the sort of rationalized work ethic that shaped modern capitalism. According to Weber, the English Puritans, in particular, had an ambivalent attitude toward the accumulation of wealth. On the one hand, he described their attitude as one that saw "riches as such [as] a great danger, their temptations unremitting, the effort to acquire them not only senseless when compared with the surpassing importance of the Kingdom of God, but also morally hazardous."

Yet the Puritans had no fundamental objection to riches, as long as they were enjoyed (or perhaps more accurately, were not enjoyed) in the right spirit. For this brand of Protestantism, Weber wrote,

> The real object of moral condemnation is, in particular, relaxation in the possession of property and enjoyment of riches, resulting in sloth and the lusts of the flesh, and above all in distraction from the pursuit of the "holy" life. And it is only because possessions bring with them the risk of this kind of relaxation that they are hazardous . . . Man must, if he is to be sure of being in a state of grace, "work the works of Him that sent him, while it is day." Not sloth and enjoyment, but only activity . . . serves to increase [God's] glory.

For the Puritans, Weber argued, "to rest content on the riches which one has already gained nearly always presaged moral failure." Weber emphasized the importance to the Puritans of the idea that everyone in society had a particular "calling," that is, a vocation toward which God had ordained he or she must work. And the riches that were often the natural consequence of working at one's proper vocation with a devoted heart were "only dangerous as a temptation to idle repose and sinful enjoyment of life, and the endeavor to acquire them was only suspect when its purpose was to enable one later to live a life of frivolity and gaiety."

Weber's great insight was that certain forms of Protestantism developed a concept of the ascetic life in which a sanctifying denial of the body's desires, far from mandating a retreat from the world in the manner of monks or hermits, actually encouraged the rationalization of work in general, and the accumulation of capital in particular. To accumulate ceaselessly, but to refuse to be seduced by the temptations inherent in enjoying the fruits of that accumulation, was the key to salvation—as was the ability to defer gratification in the pursuit of a sanctified soul. Indeed, these things—for the English Puritans whose beliefs would end up having such a profound impact on American culture—were signs of election, by which all might know just whom God, in His omniscience, had elected for admission into the Kingdom of Heaven.

What does all this have to do with the obsession so many contemporary Americans have with fat, food, and body image? After all, contemporary America is a highly secularized culture, at least in comparison to the society in which the Puritan thinkers whose works Weber interprets lived and wrote. When modern Americans labor to accumulate, surely it is not because they believe that driving a luxury car or living in an enormous house are signs of spiritual election (although ideas along such lines can certainly still be found among branches of evangelical Protestantism). Yet if we look closely, we will find much in Weber's analysis of the relationship between seventeenth-century Protestant ideology and social structures it helped shape that still applies to the America of today.

Consider the implications of the fact that in contemporary America thinness and fatness correlate well with upper- and lower-class status, respectively. Now on one level this phenomenon has little to do with the particular conditions of American social and economic life. We can predict that thinness will come to be considered desirable in societies where food is cheap and abundant for the same reason that fatness is considered desirable in societies where food is scarce and expensive: because, in each case, the desirable characteristic is difficult to achieve for those to whom it does not come naturally, and therefore possessing it tends to become identified with the possession of social rank and privilege.

An amusing, if rather depressing, example of this is provided by many passages in Susan Estrich's *Making the Case for Yourself*: passages in which she acknowledges that, for women such as herself (that is, women whose natural weight is 20 or so pounds above the cultural ideal), maintaining thinness is an expensive proposition. For example, she advises those of her readers "who can possibly afford it" to hire a personal trainer, and then, apparently recognizing the awkward sorts of socioeconomic (and therefore political) issues this sort of suggestion raises, she relates a story whose purpose is to confirm her middle-class credentials. One year for her birthday, she tells her readers, she asked her husband for a trainer. She adds that the trainer "charges a lot less than most 'Hollywood trainers,'" but then acknowledges, "I know a good many people can't afford that." She adds that, "I probably can't afford it. I shop at Ross and Loehmann's and Filene's Basement. But I also have a personal trainer. I figure I wear my body."

Like many upper-class people, Estrich talks as if she has no idea how much money the average American actually lives on. Without getting into trade secrets, suffice it to say that a senior law professor at the University of Southern California who also writes a fairly successful nationally syndicated column surely makes at least $250,000 per year from those two sources alone, making her "I shop at discount clothing stores" routine ring rather hollow to anyone with a clue regarding what her tax forms must look like.

None of this keeps Estrich from sharing such insights as, "Why does Sharon Stone always look so great? Reportedly, she has a great chef who cooks healthy meals for her made of all the things she likes. Nothing wrong with that." (Now there's a diet plan the average American can really use.) Or, "the next time you get incredibly angry and are ready to eat everything in sight, go get your nails done (always a sure-fire food stopper)." As Estrich emphasizes repeatedly, for tens of millions of Americans, staying thin either is or would be a full-time job. Yet it's also the kind of full-time job that you have to pay a lot of money to perform, as opposed to the kind that pays you to do it. It is, in other words, the sort of thing that isn't easy to afford, which helps explain why, for people such as Estrich, thinness has become a species of luxury good, the possession of which is closely identified with upper-class status.

Nevertheless, in America today the identification of thinness with social privilege—and ultimately with virtue—goes well beyond the more or less universal economic fact that things that are difficult to acquire tend to become desirable almost by default. In an important sense, the logic of contemporary consumer capitalism finds its purest expression in the diet culture. Consider that consumer capitalism depends in large part on the ability to regularly exacerbate our sense of desire. As consumers, we must be constantly hungering for "more," whatever more might be. A satisfied consumer ceases to consume, until he is no longer satisfied: Thus a kind of institutionalized sense of recurrent dissatisfaction is critical to the health and expansion of consumer markets.

The implications of this for the culture of food and fat obsession are stark but clear. Part of what disgusts the thin rich about the fat poor is the failure of the latter to recognize that hunger is, in the broadest sense, a virtue. In regard to this point, Weber's insights about the nature of the Protestant work ethic and the spirit of capitalism are particularly germane. To labor ceaselessly to acquire, without ever allowing oneself to indulge in the satisfaction that such acquisition might otherwise bring, is, within the context of this ideology, the mark of the elect ("to rest content in the riches one has already gained presages moral failure)."

It is striking that the similarities between, on the one hand, Weber's description of the Protestant work ethic, and, on the other, the contemporary American diet ethic have gone largely unnoticed. In each case the road to virtue, and to eventual election—defined as the salvation of the soul in the former instance, and the apotheosis of the body in the latter—is to labor ceaselessly at a task that can never be completed, while perpetually deferring gratification in the pursuit of an ideal that, as an axiomatic matter in the case of Protestant theology, and a practical one in the case of dieting dogma, can never be achieved on this earth. (The main difference between the two is that while it remains possible the believer may one day be united with the communion of saints, it is not actually possible for the dieter to ever lose "the last 10 pounds" that will produce the bodily apotheosis the priests of dieting promise to their ever-trusting flocks.)

More specifically, in America today, the ability to control one's food impulses has become associated with the ability to control and sublimate desire in general, but most particularly with the ability to control all aspects of one's job, finances, and economic interests. As Greg Critser notes, "in upscale corporate America, being fat is a sure-fire career-killer. If you can't control your own contours, goes the logic, how can you control a budget and staff?" (As we saw, the absurdity of this "logic" did not deter Critser himself from accepting its validity.)

Yet underneath the absurd generalization that an ability to stick to a diet is a good proxy for possessing the kind of self-discipline valued by employers (as Estrich's dieting autobiography demonstrates, it's just as likely that periods of weight gain would correlate with times of high achievement, since the non-dieter would be putting all of her energies into her job, rather than her diet) there still lurks a grain of truth, which the cult of dieting exaggerates into a whole series of claims about the relationship between thinness and virtue. After all, few things could represent the ability to defer gratification—the ability that Weber and many others have identified as the bourgeois value par excellence—than the ability to stay perpetually 20 pounds under whatever weight genetics and environment predispose a person to maintain.

People can be thin for many reasons. In cultures in which involuntary starvation is rare, the most common reason will always be that certain individuals are inclined genetically to maintain slender figures. Still, a significant number of Americans manage to maintain lower weight levels than they would otherwise enjoy through efforts of will that last years, and in some cases decades. (On the other hand, as the dominant culture grows increasingly intolerant of any sort of body diversity, and the definition of slenderness gets ratcheted constantly downward, more and more people who were previously thin no longer are, even if they haven't gained any weight.) Even though the vast majority of dieters fail to maintain long-term weight loss, there are still going to be millions of "successful" dieters in a nation where roughly 115 million Americans are dieting at any one time. Furthermore, there are large numbers of people—no one knows just how many—who don't formally diet but who are nevertheless acculturated to behaving in a manner that leaves them thinner than they would be otherwise, if they ate normally and exercised moderately. In a sense, these people have never been on a diet because they have never really been off one.

Thus the aristocracy of thinness in America today is made up of two overlapping classes: the naturally thin, and those who have achieved an unnatural thinness (in other words, thinness represents either genetic luck, or some combination of individual willpower and social privilege sufficient to produce whatever the culture defines as

thinness in a particular individual's case). And, in a society in which
"health" and "wellness" have become secular equivalents to the Puritan concept of sanctification through work, it was perhaps inevitable
that what began almost a century ago as the idea that thinness was
fashionable has metamorphosed gradually into the belief that thinness
was not merely a matter of fashion but rather a mark of virtue. It is no
coincidence that obesity research has spent much of this time "prov-
ing" that thinness is necessary to health. For it is precisely this sham
discovery that has allowed thinness to become not merely a proxy for
the ability to work ceaselessly at an unending task, and a mark of a
willingness to defer gratification, but a necessary condition for entering into the secular equivalent of a state of grace. (A striking example
of the urge to transform health issues into matters of moral choice is
provided by the reaction of an author of a recent study finding that
people who live to be one hundred have larger than average cholesterol-
carrying molecules. "I hate to say it," he said, "but if you have this gene
you can smoke and you can be fat and you can not exercise. This sounds
terrible to me.")

Ultimately the war on fat is both a cause and a consequence of the
transformation of the Protestant work ethic into the American diet
ethic. The intense hold the cult of thinness exercises over our culture,
reflected in that cult's ability to squelch attempts to discuss rationally
such issues as the relationship between weight and health, is in large
part enabled by the mostly invisible ideological power the American
diet ethic wields. And much of that power springs from the curious
historical process by which the virtues of the Protestant work ethic,
and all the advantages for the practice of consumer capitalism those
virtues entail, have been transmogrified into the virtues of thinness.

"Man," wrote Dostoyevsky, "cannot exist without bowing before
something. Let him reject God and he will bow before an idol." The
things many Americans worship today—"health," "fitness," a perpetually youthful body—have become so closely associated with staying or
becoming thin that, for all practical purposes, what such people worship is a god of perpetual slenderness. For them, weight control has
become the equivalent of that sanctifying avocation Weber's Puritan
theologians believed every individual was obligated to seek. Which
brings us at last to the connection between anorexia nervosa and the
spirit of capitalism.

On its face, the obesity myth is a product of a simple and cynical

swindle. The weight loss industry exploits cultural anxieties about fat
to sell its customers products that don't work, over and over again, by
convincing those customers that it is *they* who are defective. The failure of these products is ascribed to the moral weakness of those who
purchase them, thus allowing the cycle to go on indefinitely. But the
situation is more complex than this. It takes a great deal of cultural
distortion to cause normal market mechanisms to break down so completely (blaming your customers for the catastrophic failure of your
products isn't usually considered a sound business practice).

The obesity myth thrives in contemporary America because America
is an eating-disordered culture. Moreover, the prime symptoms of this
situation—our increasing rates of "overweight," bulimia, and anorexia—
are also symptoms of, and have become metaphors for, a broader set of
cultural anxieties.

Americans worry, with good reason, that we have become too big
for our own good: that we consume too much, too quickly; that our
cars, our houses, and our shopping malls are too large; that our impe-
rial ambitions to make the world safe for democracy and McDonald's
(not necessarily in that order) are too grand. Under these circumstances, obsessing about the 10 pounds of "extra" weight that the
average American adult has gained over the last fifteen years has become a convenient way of avoiding a more direct engagement with any
number of issues regarding America's size, excessiveness, and out-of-
control consumption.

One way of understanding America's current obsession with "obesity" is as a symptom of a deeper fear that we are threatening to consume the entire planet. Bulimia, for example, can be taken as a good
metaphor for the excesses of consumer capitalism. As long ago as the
1950s, marketing analyst Victor Lebow pointed out that "our enormously productive economy demands that we make consumption a
way of life, that we convert the buying and use of goods into rituals,
that we seek our spiritual satisfaction in consumption . . . We need
things consumed, burned up, worn out, replaced, and discarded at an
ever-increasing rate." In such a culture, the binge-purge rituals of bu-
limics mirror our acquisitive frenzy, in which we purchase far more
than we need, only to purge ourselves as a host of new items is added
to consumer capitalism's endless buffet, in its doomed quest to satisfy
our insatiable appetites.

For upper-class Americans in particular, it's easier to deal with anxiety about excessive consumption by obsessing about weight, rather than by actually confronting far more serious threats to our social and political health. Upper-class Americans are much thinner than their working-class and poor brethren, and they consume much more. (In America today there is an inverse relationship between body size and income, and income levels largely determine overall levels of consumption.) We may drive environmentally insane SUVs that dump untold tons of hydrocarbons into the atmosphere; we may consume a vastly disproportionate share of the world's diminishing natural resources; we may support a foreign policy that consists of throwing America's military weight around without regard to objections from our allies— but at least we don't eat that extra cookie when it's offered to us.

All of which is to say that the current panic over fat is in part a traditional search for societal scapegoats. Indeed, as UCLA sociologist Abigail Saguy suggested to me, our current hysteria about weight can be understood as a moral panic. "Moral panic" is a term coined by Stanley Cohen in the 1960s to describe a recurrent social pattern. First, a group or behavior is classified as dangerously deviant. The deviance is characterized as both a serious threat to societal welfare and as a symptom of deep social ills. The media whips up public concern on the subject by focusing rapidly increasing amounts of attention on it, often in an alarmist fashion that exaggerates the extent of—and the danger presented by—the behavior and those who engage in it. This in turn leads decision makers to act, usually with the stated goal of completely eliminating, or at least greatly reducing, the deviants and/or their behavior. Whether or not the action is successful, the panic eventually recedes as public attention moves on to other threats, real or imagined.

American history is rich with examples of moral panics. From witchcraft trials in colonial Massachusetts, to nineteenth-century anxieties about immigrants, urban criminals, and freed slaves, to twentieth-century panics over communists in the State Department, violence in our schools, satanic cultists in our day care centers, and the more or less perennial panic over the demonic triad of sex, drugs, and rock and roll, no period of American history has been immune to the widespread belief that the health and morals of the people in general, and of our youth in particular, have degenerated from what they were in the (largely mythical) past. It is no coincidence that our moral panic over weight is focused on what Greg Critser calls "the deadly fattening of our youth." Nor is it a coincidence that, amid America's whirlwind of overconsumption, with its attendant anxieties about our economic, cultural, and military voraciousness, our anorexic Puritans promise that we can maintain our virtue by refusing to surrender to the most literal of our gluttonous impulses.

As many people have pointed out, the classic symptoms of anorexia—refusing to maintain normal body weight, denying the dangers that accompany self-starvation, a terror of being "fat," engaging in compulsive rituals in regard to eating, dividing all food into "good" and "bad" categories—are all, at bottom, part of the ordinary day-to-day mental state of people living their lives in the diet culture. The anorexic merely takes the logic of that culture to an often deadly extreme (anorexia has a higher fatality rate than any other mental illness). In her pursuit of virtue, she becomes a secularized shadow of the so-called holy anorexics of premodern Europe: women in the grip of religious enthusiasms who would mortify their bodies by starving themselves, or by other means, such as ingesting disgusting substances. The unholy anorexic of America's secularized work ethic merely demonstrates in particularly sharp relief that, for those who worship the god of slenderness, their bodies are their work, with "work" here being both a noun and verb. That is, their bodies are both their vocation and the ongoing, never perfected product of that vocation.

What is the anorexic, in the end, but the perfect dieter? Nothing demonstrates her virtue better than the fact that she is *always working*, working ceaselessly; and that she defers the sordid pleasures of mere bodily gratification far more completely (except on those rare occasions when she is forced to eat) than the half-hearted adepts who are constantly going "on" and "off" their diets. She is, in a word, both the perfect worker and the perfect consumer, both because her labor never ends, and because she can never be satisfied, given that what she wants to consume is nothing less than her very self. Her entire life is devoted to achieving election by ridding herself utterly of vice, in the form of fat, and replacing it with a virtuous nothingness, with an unbearable lightness of being, that cannot be granted her in this life.

Anorexics understand this well, which is why so many anorexic websites (these are sites dedicated to helping anorexics continue being anorexic) have sprung up on the Internet—hundreds, at last count. And indeed, given the logic of the diet culture—given our culture's profound fear and loathing of fat and its identification of an ever-thinner bodily ideal with the most virtuous vocation that can be pursued while paying homage to the god of perpetual slenderness—who can blame the anorexic for taking things just one tiny (size less-than-zero?) step further? Like Kafka's hunger artist, why should she stop now, when she is in her best fasting form, or rather, not quite yet in her best fasting form?

If the thin are the elect, has she not proven her virtue more fully than anyone else? If fat disgusts, is she not the least disgusting of those who, in this world at least, remain cursed with the burden of gross corporeality? If "by their works ye shall know them," then the anorexic's emaciated body, hardly distinguishable though it now is from that of the average fashion model or movie star, is nothing less than the masterwork of the diet culture. Indeed, is not her body in its own way the clearest sign of virtue, the most unimpeachable evidence of election, that the culture of fat hatred could hope to look upon, with horror, with envy, and with the shock of recognition?

18

The Last American Diet

NEAR THE END OF HIS ESSAY "Why I Write" George Orwell makes the following observation:

> Looking back through the last page or two, I see that I have made it appear as though my motives in writing were wholly public-spirited. I don't want to leave that as the final impression. All writers are vain, selfish and lazy, and at the very bottom of their motives there lies a mystery. Writing a book is a horrible, exhausting struggle, like a long bout of some painful illness. One would never undertake such a thing if one were not driven on by some demon whom one can neither resist nor understand. For all one knows, that demon is simply the same instinct that makes a baby squall for attention. And yet it is also true that one can write nothing readable unless one constantly struggles to efface one's personality.

Looking back through the last three hundred pages, I feel the truth behind Orwell's words. Indeed my own motives in writing this book were far from wholly public-spirited. Besides the usual assortment of desires that plague the narcissistic tribe of writers—to be the center of attention, to be admired for one's cleverness, to make money without having to get out of one's chair—I was also driven by something else.

Grappling with the meaning of this further motive is something I would prefer to avoid altogether, as it is both a painful subject and one that I'm far from fully understanding. But it can no longer be avoided.

When I read over this manuscript I'm struck by how often it seems to imply that its author, unlike most of the people he criticizes, has achieved a healthy, well-balanced attitude toward questions of food, fat, and body image. Indeed, without ever exactly having intended to do so I realize now that, by leaving my own story out of the equation, I've given the reader what in many ways is a false impression. So let me reveal a few things about myself that are relevant to this whole topic and that I've avoided discussing up to this point.

When I began to write this book I was fat. A height of 5'8" combined with a weight of 215 pounds made me, according to the federal government, solidly "obese." Now, four years later, I weigh 160 pounds and inhabit the blessed realm of those with supposedly "ideal" BMI figures between 19 and 24.9. How did this happen, and why? I have a much better sense of the answer to the first question than the second one.

Throughout childhood and adolescence I was always a bit on the heavy side. I wasn't fat, exactly—just somewhat chubbier than the average kid. No doubt if I had been a girl I would have been considered fat, period. As a boy I was what was often called "stocky." In high school I weighed barely more than I do today, when even by the obsessive standards of this culture many people would consider me thin: But of course 165 pounds looks very different on a teenage boy than it does on a forty-three-year-old man. In any case, I had a perhaps more than ordinarily miserable time in high school: My family moved to a different city the summer before tenth grade, and for whatever combination of reasons I became antisocial and depressed. I made no new friends, I never went out anywhere, and by my senior year I was on the verge of flunking out of school, which, given that I attended a public high school in the mid-1970s, was a rather remarkable achievement in its own right.

All this began to change in the middle of my senior year when—God only knows how—I acquired a girlfriend: a 5-foot-tall, 90-pound waif who in retrospect resembled a sort of pre-Raphaelite version of Winona Ryder. This romance turned my life around in various ways, not the least significant of which took place when, several months after we became a couple, she mentioned as tactfully as she could that I could stand to lose 10 pounds. Taken aback, but feeling in no position to argue, I started jogging, cut back on midnight snacks, and began drinking a particularly vile diet soda called "Tab," the sight of a can of which will, for me, always conjure the 1970s as surely as the whiff of marijuana smoke or the sounds of KC & the Sunshine Band.

With a teenager's metabolism on my side I shed 35 pounds in a matter of three or four months, and reached a weight of 130 pounds, which, even allowing for my age, was an extremely low figure for someone with my basic build. I still remember the distinct thrill I got the day I looked at myself in a full-length mirror and realized that the mildly plump boy I had always been had transformed himself into a genuinely thin fellow. I also remember the insight that broke upon me like a Joycean epiphany when, not long after, my girlfriend asked me to stop running so much, as it was making my thighs too thick (I owe her a great deal, and I'm aware this narrative is making her seem vain and superficial, which for the most part she was not).

Anyway, I spent the bulk of my twenties as what might be called a fat person in a thin body. That is, although no one would have considered me fat, my mental self-image was that of a fat person who was "passing" as thin. Therefore, although I never formally dieted, I remained very conscious of what I ate, and I continued to jog regularly, strictly for "fitness" purposes—meaning weight maintenance (at that time I never entered races, or had any interest in participating in the competitive sport of running per se). Looking back, I realize now that I associated being "fat" with the misery and loneliness of my first two years of high school, and that I must have feared becoming fat again. Even so, in the natural course of events I gained weight over the decade, to the point where I weighed about 170 pounds as I entered my thirties. My frame had filled out, so I wasn't nearly as "fat" at this weight as I had been at a similar weight fifteen years earlier. Still, I was no longer thin when, shortly after my thirty-first birthday, my first wife filed for divorce.

Over the course of the next several months I followed the same routine: I would go jogging in the morning on an empty stomach and then generally eat nothing until the evening, when I would consume something along the lines of five large Entenmann's chocolate doughnuts. This extremely unhealthy routine led me to shed 25 pounds quite quickly. I also became fairly depressed. Only after establishing a stable relationship with another woman did I return to normal eating patterns, partially in response to the fact that she kept pointing out that a willingness to maintain a diet of five Entenmann's chocolate doughnuts indicated a less than healthy attitude toward food.

After we married, and especially after the birth of our daughter, my weight began to climb again. Over the course of my mid- and late thirties I must have gained an average of around 6 to 8 pounds per year, although I've never owned a scale, and thus would often go for months or even a year or two without weighing myself. The quantity and speed of my jogging also declined, to the point where I was jogging a dozen twelve-minute miles per week (in other words, an adequate quantity for health purposes, but not nearly enough to have much effect on my gradual weight gain). In any case, by the fall of 1999, when I both turned forty and began to work on this book in earnest, I weighed approximately 50 pounds more than I had seven years earlier.

At this point two things happened that, in retrospect, were closely connected: My wife filed for a separation, and I once again began to lose a lot of weight. Over the course of the next year I worked furiously on this book, started running farther and faster, went to marriage counseling, reconciled with my wife, and lost 67 pounds, hitting a low of 148 pounds at the beginning of 2001. Now, in the winter of 2004, I find myself still married, still thin (by the standards of most cultures, that is, although not this one, whose government would label me "overweight" if I gained 5 pounds), and still angry and confused about what all this means. To return to the question with which I began this chapter: How and why did I lose 30% of my body mass in the course of writing a book whose central purpose is to document the fundamental dishonesty and injustice of the war on fat?

The "how" is relatively straightforward: After an initial period of depression brought on by a crisis in my personal life, I became conscious of a change in my eating habits, and I gradually upped the quantity and quality of my running. I never dieted—that is, I never counted calories, kept a food journal, or cut any particular food out of my diet completely—but I did become much more aware of just what I was eating and when. I also ended up increasing my running from twelve miles per week of slow jogging to around forty miles per week of fairly focused training for road races, which I began to enter for the first time in my life. Losing weight was a necessary but far from sufficient condition for transforming myself from a fitness jogger into a competitive runner, albeit one who competes essentially against

himself. Nevertheless, by the fall of 2001 I was taking great pride in
finishing among the top 15% or so of most of the races I entered—as a
classic last-kid-picked-in-gym-class, I had never before managed to
achieve mediocrity in any athletic event, so even this modest level of
athletic success meant a great deal to me. Thus by a combination of
becoming more aware of what I was eating and greatly increasing my
level of physical activity I had transformed myself from solidly fat to
something like thin.

Yet even as I read over these words I wonder to what extent I'm
mischaracterizing my own behavior. After all, now that I've put it down
on paper, I have to admit that my weight biography looks very much
like that of the classic yo-yo dieter. Yet I keep insisting that I haven't
dieted: And it's true that I haven't engaged in many of the standard
rituals of the diet culture. But at the same time I have, over the past
three years, often behaved in much the same manner as the chronic
restrained eaters I've criticized so freely in this book: denying myself
foods I wanted to eat while spending a good deal of time planning just
when I was going to eat and how much, and so on. Does this add up to
the "constant vigilance" recommended by those who advocate chronic
restrained eating? I'd like to think my own behavior has fallen well
short of that austere standard; then again, I'm surely not the best person to judge this matter. I do know that some of the passion with
which I have lashed out at the diet culture's power to convince people
to waste much of their lives pursuing an essentially empty goal is a
product of the fact that it has had that sort of power over me.

Indeed I can easily imagine an unsympathetic reader interpreting
much of this book, given its author's own experiences, as an elaborate
exercise in hypocrisy. For one thing, it doesn't take a depth psychologist to figure out that I tend to lose weight when women leave me, or
hint that they might. So there you have it: I lambasted Susan Estrich
for publishing a diet book designed to help a woman "hold her man,"
at the very same time that I was losing weight partly in reaction to
similar anxieties of my own. Does this make me a hypocrite? I suppose
on one level it does. It certainly makes me a much weaker and more
fallible human being than the imaginary figure lurking behind the confident, quasi-omniscient voice in which a good deal of this book is
written.

Furthermore, I don't doubt that spending several years studying
how badly fat people are treated in America is a terrific incentive to

lose weight. As a fat person who currently inhabits a thin body, it both angers and saddens me to consider how much work I myself have devoted to "passing"—for that is what being thin always feels like to those of us who grew up anything like fat. As much as I despise the message of self-hatred that, as one of my correspondents put it, every fat person in America is taught to believe, I seem to have internalized that message quite effectively. I like myself more when I'm thin— not because I'm healthier (I was in excellent overall health when I weighed 55 pounds more than I do at present), or because I'm now a better human being in any way that actually matters, but because people treat me as if I were a more admirable person when I'm thin rather than fat, and I do not have the psychic strength to resist that insidious message.

To be painfully honest about the matter, I loved the compliments I got from people (usually women) about my weight loss. Coworkers who hadn't said a thing to me when I received various professional honors couldn't stop asking me how I had "done it." Indeed, I became sufficiently addicted to these comments that, when I realized some people were hesitating to say anything because they knew something about my book's thesis, I became increasingly annoyed. "Go ahead," I wanted to say, "it's okay to tell me how great I look." It's terribly embarrassing to admit these sorts of things (physical vanity is considered less forgivable in men than in women), but a candid accounting of my own experiences demands it.

All of which is to say that recognizing the injustice of something does not necessarily rob that thing of its power over oneself. If this book reads like an indictment of the diet culture, that's because it is— and one of the things that makes me angriest about that culture is that a part of me remains so firmly in its grip. Indeed, sometimes I ask myself if part of my motive for writing this book was to make myself thinner by intellectualizing the whole issue, in something of the manner of a novelist who manages to quit smoking by writing a novel about a character who spends his life trying to quit smoking. (In a Borges-like twist that would have pleased Italo Svevo, Richard Klein managed to quit smoking by writing a book—*Cigarettes Are Sublime*—about Svevo's novel based on that very premise.)

And, as the previous sentence attests, even now I find myself intellectualizing issues that, as I have noted several times when referring to other people's problems, are often too painful to face straightforwardly.

How then should I interpret my own weight loss? Am I a normally fat person who, by engaging in far more strenuous exercise than necessary to maintain optimum health, has managed to make himself into someone of "abnormally average" weight? Or am I a normally average-weight person who, precisely because he grew up in a culture that condemns fat so ferociously and irrationally, ended up becoming abnormally fat? I'm far too close to these matters to be able to answer such questions with confidence, but for what it's worth I believe the truth lies somewhere in the middle. That is, I don't think I would have ever weighed as much as 215 pounds in a culture that had a more rational attitude toward weight, but I also suspect that, if I lived in such a culture, I would weigh more than I do at present.

Still, I don't want to oversimplify. Although, to echo Orwell, my motives for writing this book were far from wholly public-spirited, I believe that, in struggling with these issues, I've managed to glimpse the beginning of wisdom regarding these matters (not that I've discovered any truth that many others before me hadn't already found, but each of us must tell his or her own story). Over the course of the past four years, in both good and bad ways, I've reconnected with my body as well as with my feelings about food and the anxieties that these subjects raise. Weight loss driven by a self-hatred born of the culture's fear and loathing of fat is clearly not a good thing, nor is it something that is likely to last. On the other hand, that is only part of the story of my own weight loss, and, no doubt, of that experienced by many others.

In the course of working on this book I've sometimes imagined I've caught a glimpse of another country. In this land, weight loss, when it took place, would be a by-product of developing healthier attitudes toward food and fitness rather than a goal in and of itself. Weight loss, in such a land, would be considered a positive thing to the extent it gave evidence that people were pursuing healthier lives in general. In such a country it would be recognized that many heavier-than-average people already live healthy lives, and that most people who change their eating and exercise habits for the better lose little or no weight. In other words, a society that maintained a rational attitude toward weight would treat being fat (or thin) as no more than what it is: a human characteristic fairly meaningless in itself, which some people find attractive, and others don't. In such a land the idea of condemning people for their weight would be considered as absurd as condemning people for their height or for the color of their skin.

I also believe that, in such a country, people would find it a good deal easier to lose weight than they do in our own culture, because losing (or not losing) weight would be considered a trivial thing. Perhaps, then, the last American diet—the one diet that would actually "work"—is that (anti)diet that would grasp the almost Zen-like character of this truth: If weight is not an issue, then weight will not be an issue. If you want to achieve a healthy weight, stop wanting to lose weight and start wanting those things—an active life, good food, and the calm enjoyment of both—that, unlike weight loss, are unalloyed goods in and of themselves. If you can manage to do this, you may well lose weight in the process; but far more important, you will get to a place where the weight you lose has been lost precisely because you no longer care, at some deep level of self-acceptance, whether you've lost weight or not.

If we Americans could somehow collectively reach that place, we might, ironically, become a good deal thinner than we are now. In a culture that accepted rather than demonized fat, people would find it much easier to eat well and be physically active than they do in America today, where these things are seen as tools for undertaking an often futile task, rather than as ways of living whose value is quite independent of whether they lead to weight loss or not.

I certainly haven't reached that place myself. The passages in this book that sound as if they were written by a supremely self-assured author, who has all the answers to our profound national neurosis regarding these matters, are in their own way as misleading as anything one can find in the obesity literature. After all, it appears my own journey toward a land where we accept our bodies for what they are has barely begun. Maybe we'll meet there some day.

> Failing to fetch me at first keep encouraged
> Missing me one place search another,
> I stop somewhere waiting for you.
> —Walt Whitman

Conclusion

WHAT THEN IS TO BE DONE? Those of us who question the current orthodoxy about weight in America deal routinely with the objection that we are "giving people permission to be fat." It's always tempting to reply to this with another question: As opposed to what—*not* giving people permission to be fat? We've been employing that particular strategy for about one hundred years now, and it has made us both the fattest people in the developed world, and increasingly miserable about the fact. If medical science has established anything it is this: In a nation in which food is cheap and plentiful, and in which it is easy to become sedentary, telling people they should lose weight by eating less and exercising more *does not work*. The blindness of the public health establishment to this astonishingly obvious point is one of the most remarkable features of the war on fat. Indeed, by now the single proposition that has been best established about the relationship between social policy and weight is that, if you want to produce a culture full of fat people, you ought to do exactly what the medical establishment and the government have been doing in America for a century now, which is to medicalize and moralize the issue of fat through a series of increasingly hysterical pronouncements about the evils of "excess" weight. Much as in the case of the drug war, the establishment's reaction to all this is to demand that we keep doing what we've been doing, only more so, apparently on the basis of the belief that a policy that produced one outcome over the course of the twentieth century will produce precisely the opposite outcome, if we just have the discipline to stick with it for another one hundred years.

The perverse paradox at the heart of the obesity myth is that this myth creates exactly what it most fears and loathes. At the core of that fear and loathing lies an especially transitory aesthetic judgment: a judgment both generated and supported by a mass of half-conscious prejudices about what "fat" supposedly tells us. In a culture that pays a good deal of lip service to egalitarian values, fat prejudice allows the traditional disgust that the rich have felt for the poor, that white people have felt for the darker-skinned, that gentiles have felt for Jews, and so forth, to be expressed indirectly, through a sanctimonious (and largely false) judgment about the terrible things "those people" are doing to their health by allowing themselves to get so fat. Fat people, according to this set of myths, are dirty, lazy, undisciplined, lustful, impulsive, and so on. That is, they display all the characteristics attributed to social pariahs, no matter who those pariahs happen to be.

The crucial role the health justification for fat prejudice plays in all this is clear: Since, from this perspective, being disgusted by fat is no different than being disgusted by cowardice or criminality, the thin can be disgusted with the fat *for their own good*, since such disgust can function as a stern corrective, placing those in need of it on the road to reform and salvation. A series of arbitrary aesthetic judgments—matters of fashion, really—along with a mass of unsavory prejudices, are then buried under a blizzard of public health propaganda, and the darker impulses that fuel the war on fat need never be acknowledged.

So what *should* we do about fat in America? We shouldn't do anything about it, other than to try to stop obsessing on the subject (of course practical problems arise when one tries consciously to stop obsessing about something). The prosecutors in the case against fat aren't completely wrong: They've just indicted the wrong parties. Americans are too sedentary. We do eat too much junk that isn't good for us, because it's quick and cheap and easier than the alternative of spending the time and money to prepare food that is both good for us and satisfies our cravings. A rational public health policy would focus on those issues, not on weight, which isn't the problem, any more than diets and diet drugs would be the solution, even if they actually made people thin (thin people with bad health habits are no healthier than fat people with the same habits).

Such a policy would emphasize that the keys to good health (that anyone can do anything about, that is—genetic factors remain far more important than anything else) are, in roughly descending order of importance: not to smoke, not to be an alcoholic or a drug addict, not to be sedentary, and not to eat a diet packed with junk food. It's true that a more active populace that ate a healthier diet would be somewhat thinner, as would a nation that wasn't dieting obsessively. Even so, there is no reason why there shouldn't be tens of millions of healthy, happy people of more-than-average weight in America, as there no doubt would be in a culture that maintained a rational attitude toward the fact that people will always come in all shapes and sizes, whether they live healthy lives or not.

If this had been a better book it would have had everything in it. It would have included the story about Cher canceling a magazine photo shoot not once but twice because she had gained 1 pound. It would have talked about how Calista Flockhart's publicity people, after a flurry of stories noted she was looking very much like a concentration camp victim, decided their client needed to eat a hot dog while sitting in a box at Yankee Stadium during the World Series, and how this took place at the height of the Clinton-Lewinsky scandal, and what this particular collocation of events might have meant, underneath the hype and the absurdity and the black humor of it all.

A better book would have talked about *What to Expect When You're Expecting*, the best-selling book for pregnant women, especially the passages that try to convince the reader she will give birth to a three-headed monster if she should so much as glance at a Snickers bar at any point during what could quite properly be called her confinement. It would have talked about the story Jeff Pearlman wrote for *Sports Illustrated* regarding star pitcher David Wells, that did nothing but talk about how fat Wells was, and how Pearlman wrote this just a few weeks after he had gotten John Rocker in so much trouble by reporting that Rocker had said offensive things about gays and foreigners, and just a week before *Sports Illustrated* did an eight-page soft-porn spread on Anna Kournikova, a tennis player who has never won a single professional tournament, but who has a couple of other talents that have made her the highest-paid woman in her field.

It would have quoted Rosie O'Donnell about going to her doctor for a physical. He told her, "You have to lose weight: In the morning, eat a bowl of cereal and skim milk, at lunch have a salad, and for dinner eat fish," and how she replied, "Thank you, you just cured obesity in America." It would have talked about restaurant portions, and how the marginal cost of giving people more than what they want is small in comparison to the cost of giving them less, and how perverse it is for a nation that always believes bigger is better to be shoving enormous amounts of food in people's faces while at the same time demanding they stay absurdly thin. A better book would have found a way to discuss the A&E network's episode of the program *Biography* about Susan Sarandon, in which viewers were expected to listen to Sarandon's views regarding various problematic aspects of Catholic theology for one reason, and one reason only: because Susan Sarandon is or perhaps once was a genuinely hot babe, as well as a pretty good actor, even though her grasp of the finer points of the *Summa Theologica* left something to be desired.

A better book would have talked about *The Sopranos*, and how part of the uncanny realism of that show involves casting mildly "overweight" to extremely fat actors in most of the male and even a couple of the female roles, although the fashionably thin Mafia wives spend much of their day at the gym, while their fat husbands shovel in the manicotti between murders; and it would have mentioned Paulie Walnuts' great line when he sees the two really fat made guys hanging out at the strip club ("Hey—it's a commercial for a diet program: Before . . . and *way* before!").

Most of all, a better book would have talked more about food. It would have conjured up memories of happiness: sizzling links of bratwurst bursting out of their skins on the Fourth of July grill, and good German beer in tall glasses beaded by the humid air, with the breeze off the river cutting through the midday heat carrying the torpid scent of green things growing in the rich, dark mud. It would have mentioned the *maguro* tuna at that beachside place in L.A. where everyone looked like an actor, especially the wait staff, so fresh you could still taste the ocean, and the *mole* sauce in Mexico City (what genius first dreamed of doing that with chile and chocolate?), and the indescribable subtlety of the saffron in the rice of a good paella. And cheap Indian restaurants in New York City, where the *masala*, and the *saag*, and the *tari aloo* make the concept of a happy vegetarian seem almost plausible. And Stilton and Manchego and all strong ripened cheeses eaten with fresh bread and fruit, especially the fat green grapes from the height of summer that practically explode in your mouth. And the pulled pork in Memphis and the barbecue in Kansas City and the filet mignon at Morton's that I can't eat anymore without feeling sick the next day, but it's still worth it. And the raspberry chocolate chip ice cream at Sebastian Joe's in Minneapolis, and every flavor of gelato from Naples to Milan, and plain hot fudge on two scoops of vanilla ice cream, anywhere on Earth.

A better book would have dealt at length with the sheer pleasure of eating, because perhaps the greatest damage done by the war on fat is how it poisons much of the joy that countless people would otherwise get from what may be our richest and most democratic sensual experience: the daily act of feeding ourselves and those we love.

A better book would have had all those things in it, and many others as well. Every book is a failure, because no book can actually say what its author envisioned, when it was all still feverish outlines and garbled notes and grand ambitions to change this or that aspect of our unsatisfactory world with nothing but the power of words on paper. Yet still, certain things that needed to be said were, in the end, said.

Notes

Foreword

"In 1986, an NIH consensus . . ." Ernsberger, P. NIH consensus conference on obesity: by whom and for what? *J Nutr.* 1987; 117:1164–1165.

"It did so despite presentations . . ." Andres, R., Muller, D.C., Sorkin, J.D. Long-term effects of change in body weight on all-cause mortality. A review. *Ann Intern Med.* 1993; 119:737–743.

"This idea did not catch on at the time . . ." NIH Tech Assess Conf Panel. Methods for voluntary weight loss and control. *Ann Intern Med.* 1993; 119:764–770.

"The fen-phen craze was triggered . . ." Weintraub, M., Sundaresan, P.R., Madan, M., Schuster, B., Balder, A., Lasagna, L., Cox, C. Long-term weight control study. I (weeks 0 to 34). The enhancement of behavior modification, caloric restriction, and exercise by fenfluramine plus phentermine versus placebo. *Clin Pharmacol Ther.* 1992; 51:586– 594.

"Editorials by obesity experts duly appeared . . ." Bray, G.A. Use and abuse of appetite-suppressant drugs in the treatment of obesity. *Ann Intern Med.* 1993; 119: 707–713.

"When I arrived to testify at the FDA hearing . . ." Ernsberger, P., Koletsky, R.J., Kilani, A., Viswan, G., Bedol, D.. Effects of weight cycling on urinary catecholamines: sympathoadrenal role in refeeding hypertension. *J Hypertens.* 1998; 16:2001–2005. Ernsberger, p., Koletsky, R.J., Baskin, J.Z., Collins, L.A. Consequences of weight cycling in obese spontaneously hypersensitive rats. *Am J Physiol.* 1996; 270:R864–R872. Ernsberger, P., Koletsky, R.J. Weight cycling. *JAMA.* 1995; 273:998–999.

"Indeed, long-term human studies show . . ." Lissner, L., Odell, P.M., D'Agostino, R.B., Stokes, J., III, Kreger, B..E, Belanger, A.J., Brownell, K.D. Variability of body weight and health outcomes in the Framingham population. *N Engl J Med.* 1991;324:1839–1844.

Chapter 1

" *'Let's look at a threat that is very real . . .'* " "Obesity Is America's Greatest Threat, Surgeon General Says," *Orlando Sentinel,* January 22, 2003, p. B1.

"From C. Everett Koop . . ." *The Dallas Morning News,* April 8, 2001, p. 1J. For Satcher's views on obesity, see *The Surgeon General's Call to Action to Prevent and Decrease Overweight and Obesity* (2001).

"Medical researchers have gone so far as to . . ." For a recent suggestion by a prominent obesity researcher that certain foods be taxed, see "Cancer Group Tries to Link Fat, Cancer in Public Mind," www.cnn.com/2003/HEALTH/diet.fitness/ 02/19cancer.weigh.in.ap/index.html (accessed February 23, 2003).

" *'A strong international consensus among scientists . . .'* " *The New Republic,* February 15, 2003 (letter).

" *'[L]ike a bad case of the flu.'* " Greg Critser, "Let Them Eat Fat," *Harper's,* March 2000, p. 42.

"According to Yale Medical School professor Kelly Brownell . . ." *Boston Globe,* May 29, 2003, p. A13.

" *'Adults should try to maintain a body mass index between 18.5 and 21.9 . . .'* " Field et al. "Impact of Overweight on the Risk of Developing Common Chronic Diseases During a 10-Year Period," *Arch Intern Med* 161, 1581–86 (2001).

"Many of the most prominent figures in obesity research have direct ties . . ." For a detailed discussion of the links between obesity researchers and the weight loss industry, see Laura Fraser, *Losing It: False Hopes and Fat Profits in the Diet Industry* (1998), pp. 209–33.

"These surgeries remain both highly profitable and extremely dangerous . . ." "Almost 2% of the patients undergoing gastric bypass surgery for morbid obesity will die within the first 30 days, according to a report presented October 21st [2003] at the American College of Surgeons 2003 Clinical Congress." Abstract from the ACS 2003 Clinical Congress.

"As University of Virginia professor Glenn Gaesser points out . . ." Glenn Gaesser, *Big Fat Lies: The Truth About Your Weight and Your Health* (2002), pp. 44–51.

"Anti-fat warriors still cite the insurance charts . . ." See, for example, Michael Fumento, "Quit Living in the Fat Lane," *Washington Times,* June 30, 2002, p. B-5. Fumento's obsession with the supposedly deadly effects of "excess" weight, illustrated by his voluminous journalism on the subject, is a particularly interesting example of the distorting effects this topic has on many media figures. In other contexts, Fumento has been at the forefront of those who denounce the distortion of public health information and agendas by ideological factors. For instance, his book *The Myth of Heterosexual AIDS* exposed how statistics are manipulated by government agencies to foment concern about a largely imaginary "epidemic." More recently, his writings regarding the panic over SARS have struck the same note. Yet when the subject is fat, the very same agencies that Fumento elsewhere treats with well-warranted skepticism are presented to readers as if they were infallible sources of objective scientific knowledge.

"Here are some figures from what at the time it was compiled was the world's largest epidemiological study to date." Waaler et al., "Height, Weight and Mortality: The Norwegian Experience, *Acta Med Scanda Suppl* 679, 1–56 (1984).

"In the late 1980s, obesity researchers Paul Ernsberger and Paul Haskew undertook a comprehensive review . . ." Ernsberger and Haskew, "Health Implications of Obesity: An Alternative View," *J Obesity W Reg* 6, 67 (1987).

"A particularly compelling illustration of this point is provided by a 1996 study . . ." Troiano et al., "The Relationship Between Body Weight and Mortality: A Quantitative Analysis of Combined Information from Existing Studies," *Int J Obesity* 20, 63–75 (1996).

"For instance, the Pooling Project . . ." McGee and Gordon, "The Results of the Framingham Study Applied to Four Other U.S.-based Epidemiological Studies of Cardiovascular Disease," in *The Framingham Study: An Epidemiological Investigation of Cardiovascular Disease,* NIH Publication #76-1083 (1976).

"Another compelling example is provided by the NHANES I survey . . ." Durazo-Arvizu et al., "Mortality and Optimal Body Mass Index in a Sample of the U.S. Population," *Am J Epidemiol* 147, 739–49 (1998).

"Yet another example comes from the famous Seven Countries Study . . ." Menotti et al., "Underweight and Overweight in Relation to Mortality Among Men Aged 40–49 and 50–59 Years: The Seven Countries Study, *Am J Epidemiol* 151, 660–66 (2000).

"Let us look at four of the most cited studies for the proposition that 'overweight' is a deadly epidemic . . ." Manson et al., "Body Weight and Mortality Among Women," *N Engl J Med* 333, 677–82 (1995); Allison et al., "Annual Deaths Attributable to Obesity in the United States," *JAMA* 282, 1530–1538 (1999); Fontaine et al., Years of Life Lost to Obesity," *JAMA* 289, 187–197 (2003); Calle et al., "Overweight, Obesity, and Mortality from Cancer in a Prospectively Studied Cohort of U.S. Adults," *New Engl J Med* 348, 1625–38 (2003).

"This range includes most of the people the government now classifies as overweight and obese." For current weight levels across the U.S. population see Flegall et al., "Prevalence and Trends in Obesity Among U.S. Adults, 1999–2000," *JAMA* 288, 1723–32 (2002).

"Even massively obese men and women do not appear to be more prone to vascular disease than average." Chambless et al., "Risk Factors for Progression of Common Carotid Atherosclerosis: The Artherosclerosis Risk in Communities Study, 1987–1998," *Am J Epidemiol* 155, 38–47 (2002).

"But even here there is considerable evidence that this correlation is not necessarily a product of being fat . . ." See Gaesser, *Big Fat Lies*, pp. 59–74.

"Obese patients who have been put on very low-calorie diets . . ." Drenick et al., "Excessive Mortality and Causes of Death in Morbidly Obese Men," *JAMA* 243, 443–45 (1980).

"When the siege of Leningrad was lifted . . ." Ancel Keys et al., *Biology of Human Starvation* (1950).

"Among those who suffer from hypertension the mortality rate from the disease is two to three times lower among heavier individuals . . ." Taminga and Yoshiba, "Prognosis of Essential Hypertension: Four-year Follow-up Study of 416 Consecutively Admitted Patients," *Jap Circ J* 31, 55–59 (1967).

"Glenn Gaesser points out the potentially deadly irony . . ." Gaesser, *Big Fat Lies*, p. 62.

"Despite the obesity epidemic, these trends are continuing with no end in sight." New York Times, January 19, 2003, Sec. 1, p. 1. See also Keys, "Is There an Ideal Body Weight?" *Brit Med J* 293, 1023–24 (1986).

"Several recent studies indicate that the key to avoiding Type 2 diabetes is . . . to make lifestyle changes . . ." Lamarche et al. "Is Body Fat Loss a Determinant Factor in the Improvement of Carbohydrate and Lipid Metabolism Following Aerobic Exercise Training in Obese Women?" *Metabolism* 41, 1249–56 (1992); Barnard

et al., "Diet and Exercise in the Treatment of NIDDM," *Diabetes Care* 17, 1469–72 (1994); Tuomilehto et al., "Prevention of Type 2 Diabetes Mellitus by Changes in Lifestyle Among Subjects with Impaired Glucose Tolerance," *New Engl J Med* 344, 1343–50 (2001); Diabetes Prevention Program Research Group, "Reduction in the Incidence of Type 2 Diabetes with Lifestyle Intervention or Metformin," *New Engl J Med* 346, 393–403 (2002).

"Over the past three decades, according to Glenn Gaesser's survey of the literature . . ." For examples see Kabat and Wynder, "Body Mass Index and Lung Cancer Risk," *Am J Epidemiol* 135, 769–74 (1992); Kabat, "Aspects of the Epidemiology of Lung Cancer in Smokers and Non-Smokers in the United States," *Lung Cancer* 15, 1–20 (1996); Avons et al. "Weight and Mortality," *Lancet* 1983, 1104 (1983); van De Brandt et al. "Pooled Analysis of Prospective Studies on Height, Weight and Breast Cancer Risk," *Am J Epidemiol* 152, 514–27 (2000); Keys et al., "Serum Cholesterol and Cancer Mortality in the Seven Countries Study," *Am J Epidemiol* 121, 870–883 (1985). See generally, Gaesser, *Big Fat Lies*, at 99–102. See also Menotti, cited above.

"Other studies have shown that heavier people are less prone to suffer from cancer . . ." Nomura et al., "Body Mass Index as a Predictor of Cancer in Men, *J Nat Cancer Inst* 74, 319–23 (1985); Lee and Kolonel, "Are Body Mass Indicies Interchangeable in Measuring Obesity-Disease Associations?" *Am J Publ Hlth* 74, 376–77 (1984); Garcia-Palmieri et al., "An Apparent Inverse Relationship Between Serum Cholesterol and Cancer Mortality in Puerto Rico," *Am J Epidemiol* 114, 29–44 (1981).

"Diseases and syndromes that various medical studies indicate are less common among heavier people include . . ." Comstock et al., "Subcutaneous Fatness and Mortality," *Am J Epidemiol* 83, 548–63 (1966); Krieger et al., "An Epidemiologic Study of Hip Fracture in Postmenopausal Women," *Am J Epidemiol* 116, 141–48 (1982); Kauffmann and Brille, "Bronchial Hypersecretion, Chronic Airflow Limitation, and Peptic Ulcer," *Am Rev Resp Dis* 124, 646–49 (1981); Hooyman et al., "Fractures from Rheumatoid Arthritis: A Population-Based Study," *Arth Rheumatism* 27, 1353–61 (1984); Tverdal, "Body Mass Index and Incidence of Tuberculosis," *Eur J Resp Dis* 69, 355–62 (1986).

"How many people are aware that heavier women have much lower rates of osteoporosis . . ." Avioli, "Significance of Osteoporosis: A Growing International Health Care Problem," *Calcif Tissue Int* 49, S5–S7 (1991); Edelstein and Barrett-Connor, "Relation Between Body Size and Bone Mineral Density in Elderly Men and Women," *Am J Epidemiol* 138, 160–69 (1993); Tremollieres et al., "Vertebral Postmenopausal Bone Loss Is Reduced in Overweight Women: A Longitudinal Study in 155 Early Postmenopausal Women," *J Clin Endocrinol Metab* 77, 683–86 (1993).

" 'Epidemiology is a crude and inexact science . . .' " *New York Times,* October 11, 1995, Sec. C, p. 1.

"To understand the implications of this distinction, consider the fact that bald men die sooner . . ." This analogy was suggested to me by Paul Ernsberger.

"The standard 'sensible' recommendations to change eating habits and diligently use caloric charts . . .' " Bennett and Gurin, *The Dieter's Dilemma* (1982), p. 283.

"The vast majority of people who attempt to lose weight eventually gain all the weight they lose back." For a recent article illustrating the extent to which dieting is a significant predictor of future weight gain, see Korkeila et al., "Weight Loss

Attempts and Risk of Major Weight Gain: A Prospective Study in Finnish Adults," *Am J Clin Nutr* 70, 965–75 (1999). See also Garner and Wooley, "Confronting the Failure of Behavioral and Dietary Treatments for Obesity," *Clin Psychol Rev* 11, 729–80 (1991).

"More Americans than ever are dieting . . ." Serdula et al., "Prevalence of Attempting Weight Loss and Strategies for Controlling Weight," *JAMA* 282, 1353–58 (1999).

"Yet Glenn Gaesser notes that numerous studies . . ." Gaesser, *Big Fat Lies,* pp. 131–45.

"In the early 1990s, a major American Cancer Society study . . ." Pamuk et al., "Weight Loss and Mortality in a National Cohort of Adults, 1971–1987," *Am J Epidemiol* 136, 686–97 (1992); Pamuk et al., "Weight Loss and Subsequent Death in a Cohort of U.S. Adults," *Ann Int Med* 119, 744–48 (1993).

"A 1999 report based on the same data pool . . ." Williamson et al., "Prospective Study of Intentional Weight Loss and Mortality in Overweight White Men Aged 40–64 Years," *Am J Epidemiol* 149, 491–503 (1999).

"The only other large study to look into the question of the health effects of intentional weight loss . . ." French et al., "Prospective Study of Intentional Weight Loss and Mortality in Older Women: The Iowa Women's Health Study," *Am J Epidemiol* 149, 504–14 (1999).

"In Steven Blair's ongoing long-term longitudinal study . . ." Blair et al., "Body Weight Change, All-Cause Mortality, and Cause-Specific Mortality in the Multiple Risk Factor Intervention Trial," *Ann Int Med* 119, 749–57 (1993).

"In the ongoing Harvard Alumni Study . . ." Lee and Paffenbarger, "Change in Body Weight and Longevity," *JAMA* 268, 2045–49 (1992).

"A recent article in a magazine published by the American Association of Retired Persons . . ." See www.aarpmagazine.com/march-april.html (accessed February 24, 2003).

"Such recommendations fly in the face of a host of recent studies . . ." Wedick et al., "The Relationship Between Weight Loss and All-Cause Mortality in Older Men and Women with and Without Diabetes Mellitus: The Rancho Bernardo Study," *J Am Geriatr Soc* 50, 1810–15 (2002); Soames et al., "Body Mass Index, Weight Change, and Death in Older Adults: The Systolic Hypertension in the Elderly Program," *Am J Epidemiol* 156, 132–38 (2002); Newman et al., "Weight Change in Old Age and Its Association with Mortality," *J Am Geriatr Soc* 49, 1309–18 (2001); Singh et al., "The Effect of Menopause on the Relation Between Weight Gain and Mortality Among Women," *Menopause* 8, 314–320 (2001); Milne et al., "Protein and Energy Supplementation in Elderly People at Risk from Malnutrition," *Cochrane Database Syst Rev* CD003288 (2002).

". . . studies that indicate weight cycling is a major factor in . . . serious health problems." Hamm et al., "Large Fluctuations in Body Weight During Young Adulthood and Twenty-five Year Risk of Coronary Death in Men," *Am J Epidemiol* 129, 312–18 (1989); Iribarren et al., "Association of Weight Loss and Weight Fluctuation with Mortality Among Japanese American Men," *New Engl J Med* 333, 686–92 (1995); Lissner et al., "Body Weight Variability and Mortality in the Gothenburg Prospective Studies of Men and Women," in *Obesity in Europe*, Bjorntorp and Rossner, eds., pp. 55–60 (1989); Brownell and Rodin, "Medical, Metabolic, and Psychological Effects of Weight Cycling," *Arch Int Med* 154, 1325–31 (1994).

"Dieters as a group run up to double the risk of developing cardiovascular disease . . ." Gaesser, *Big Fat Lies,* p. 19.

"Indeed, the more often a person diets, the stronger these cravings become." Drewnowski and Holden-Wiltse, "Taste Responses and Food Preferences in Obese Women: Effects of Weight Cycling," *Int J Obesity* 16, 639–48 (1992).

". . . visceral body fat, which is far more dangerous to health than subcutaneous fat." Bouchard et al., "Genetic and Non-Genetic Determinants of Regional Fat Distribution," *Endocrine Rev* 14, 72–93 (1993).

"As Glenn Gaesser has pointed out, given what we know about relative rates of dangerous weight loss practices . . ." "Body Fat and Health: Conventional Wisdom vs. the Evidence," Keynote Speech, 2001 NAAFA Convention, August 14, 2001, Cherry Hill, NJ.

"The list of side effects from the most popular diet drugs is long." See Ernsberger and Haskew, cited above.

"A new Yale University study . . ." Kernan et al., "Phenylpropanolamine and the Risk of Hemorrhagic Stroke," *New Engl J Med* 343, 1826–32 (2000).

"Recently four prominent athletes . . ." "Ephedra Controversy Nothing New in Sports; Dietary Supplement Linked to Other Deaths," *Washington Post*, February 20, 2003, D4.

"After the FDA hearing at which its approval was temporarily blocked . . ." "Obesity Drug; After Bitter 9-Hour Debate, FDA Panel's Ruling Still Awaited," *Chicago Tribune*, September 29, 1995, A15.

". . . a highly publicized study authored by June Stevens and others . . ." Stevens et al, "The Effect of Age on the Association Between Body-Mass Index and Mortality," *New Engl J Med* 338, 1–7 (1998).

". . . a Cooper Institute study published in JAMA . . ." Blair et al., "Physical Fitness and All-Cause Mortality: A Prospective Study of Healthy Men and Women," *JAMA* 262, 2395–2401 (1989).

"Similarly, a 1999 Cooper Institute study . . ." Lee et al., "Cardiorespiratory Fitness, Body Composition, and All-Cause and Cardiovascular Disease Mortality in Men," *Am J Clin Nutr* 69, 373–80 (1999).

"A 1995 Blair study found . . ." Barlow et al., "Physical Fitness, Mortality and Obesity," *Int J Obesity* 19, S41–S44 (1995).

"As Blair himself puts it . . ." "Exercise Benefits Even Obese People," Associated Press Wire Story, July 18, 2001.

"Ralph Paffenbarger's Harvard Alumni Study . . ." Paffenbarger et al., "Physical Activity, All-Cause Mortality, and Longevity of College Alumni," *New Engl J Med* 314, 605–13 (1986).

"The Behavioral Risk Factor Surveillance System . . ." Hahn et al., "Cardiovascular Disease Risk Factors and Preventive Practices Among Adults—United States, 1994: A Behavioral Risk Factor Atlas," *MMWR* 47, 35–72 (1998).

"And a 2002 study of nearly ten thousand Puerto Rican men . . ." Crespo et al., "The Relationship of Physical Activity and Body Weight with All-Cause Mortality: Results from the Puerto Rico Heart Health Program," *AEP* 12, 543–52 (2002).

"Indeed whether people are active or sedentary . . ." A host of studies suggest that both preexisting differences in activity levels and subsequent changes to such levels have almost no relevance to variances in body mass. For example, a ten-year study of American adults found no relationship between baseline physical activity and later weight gain among men and women. See Williamson, et al., "Recreational Physical Activity and Ten-Year Weight Change in a US National Cohort," *Int J Obesity* 17, 279–86 (1993). A recent study of nearly forty thousand female health professionals found that the average weight variance between the most sedentary and

the most active women was about 1.5 BMI units, i.e., about 7 pounds. See Lee et al., "Physical Activity and Coronary Heart Disease in Women," *JAMA* 285, 1447–54 (2001). A Harvard Alumni Study of more than twelve thousand men found essentially no weight difference between highly sedentary men who expended less than 500 calories per week in exercise activities, and extremely active men who expended more than 3,000 calories per week (the average BMIs of the two groups were 24.7 and 24.4 respectively). See Sesso et al., "Physical Activity and Coronary Heart Disease in Men," *Circulation* 102, 975–80 (2000). And a new study measuring the effects of a sixteen-month exercise regimen (2,000 calories per week) on overweight and obese women observed an average total weight loss of 1 pound, i.e., one ounce per month, among those women who did not drop out of the program. See Donnelley et al., "The Midwest Exercise Trial," *Arch Int Med* 163, 1343–50 (2003).

"In short, as Glenn Gaesser points out . . ." Big Fat Lies, p. 117.
For a few representatives of the extremely extensive literature questioning the case against fat, see, for example, Gaesser, *Big Fat Lies*, cited above; Ernsberger and Haskew, cited above; Keys, *Seven Countries: A Multivariate Analysis of Death and Coronary Heart Disease* (1980); Andres, "Beautiful Hypotheses and Ugly Facts: The BMI-Mortality Association," *Obesity Res* 7, 417–19 (1999); Hilda Bruch, *Eating Disorders* (1974); Blair, articles cited above; Barrett-Conner, "Obesity, Atherosclerosis, and Coronary Artery Disease," *Ann Int Med* 103, 1010–19 (1985); Polivy and Herman, *Breaking the Diet Habit* (1993); S. Wooley and O. Wooley, "Should Obesity Be Treated at All?" in *Eating and Its Disorders*, Stunkard and Stellar, eds. (1984); Wooley and Garner, "Obesity Treatment: The High Cost of False Hope," *J Am Diet Assoc* 91, 1248–51 (1991); Ikeda et al., "A Commentary on the New Obesity Guidelines from NIH," *J Am Diet Assoc* 99, 918–19 (1999); Kim Chernin, *The Obsession* (1981); Hillel Schwartz, *Never Satisfied: A Cultural History of Diets, Fantasies and Fat* (1986); Roberta Seid, *Never Too Thin: Why Women Are at War with Their Bodies* (1989); Richard Klein, *Eat Fat* (1996); Susan Bordo, *Unbearable Weight: Feminism, Western Culture, and the Body* (1995); Laura Fraser, *Losing It*, cited above; Naomi Wolf, *The Beauty Myth* (1991); Susie Orbach, *Fat Is a Feminist Issue* (1978).

"In his book **The Culture of Fear** *. . ."* Barry Glassner, *The Culture of Fear: Why Americans Are Afraid of the Wrong Things* (1999), pp. xxvi–xxviii.

Chapter 2

"However, there is still a fifty-billion-dollar-per year industry . . ." For one calculation of the size of the American diet industry, see Fraser, *Losing It*, p. 299. The figure could be considerably higher if one were to include items such as workout equipment, subscriptions to magazines such as *Shape* and the like, that are largely devoted to weight loss, etc.

"Basically, obesity research in America is funded by the diet and drug industry . . ." See Fraser, *Losing It*, pp. 209–32 for a detailed discussion of the economics of obesity research.

"The last sentence in this hypothetical abstract illustrates what dissident obesity researcher Susan Wooley . . ." For a good summary of Wooley's views, see Wooley and Garner, "Obesity Treatment: The High Cost of False Hope," *J Am Diet Assoc* 91, 1248–51 (1991).

"My favorite is a recent study that concludes the majority of weight variance is unalterably genetic . . ." Allison and Pi-Sunyer, "Fleshing Out Obesity," *The Sciences*, May–June 1994, 38–43.

"This is in fact a fairly accurate description of the United States during the last few decades of the nineteenth century . . ." For discussions of changing standards of beauty in American culture, see Hillel Schwartz, *Never Satisfied: A Cultural History of Diets, Fantasies and Fat* (1986); Roberta Seid *Never Too Thin: Why Women Are at War with Their Bodies* (1989). For information on Lillian Russell, see Parker Morell, *Lillian Russell: The Era of Plush* (1940).

"In West Africa today, beauty pageants feature contestants that would be considered markedly 'obese' . . ." See "Bigger Is Better at 'Miss Fat South Africa' Beauty Pageant," *Jet*, May 20, 2002, p. 55.

"When one considers the extent of the damage done by the eating disorders from which at least eight million Americans currently suffer . . ." For current statistics on eating disorders in America, see the National Association for Anorexia Nervosa and Associated Disorders website, at www.anad.org.

Chapter 3

*"The cover of the March 2000 issue of **Harper's** . . ."* Critser has since expanded his thoughts on this issue into a book, *Fat Land*, that argues for a new appreciation of "the sin of gluttony." I agree with Critser that Americans have good reasons to be concerned about overconsumption in our society. The question, however, is whether the fact that Americans gained an average of 8 pounds over the course of the 1990s has as much political, environmental, and ethical significance as such facts as that our automobiles gained an average of several hundred pounds during those years.

"This essay is in many ways representative of the sort of reportage regarding weight-related issues now appearing on a daily basis . . ." A search of the Nexis database for articles published in major English-language newspapers reveals that, as of September 2003, the claim that fat kills three hundred thousand Americans per year had appeared in more than 1,700 stories over the past two years alone.

"An outbreak of influenza in 1918 killed between twenty and forty million people . . ." See Alfred Crosby's *America's Forgotten Pandemic: The Influenza of 1918* for an account of a real epidemic, and the genuine public health crisis it engendered.

"They will never be given a hint of the fact that, in the words of the editors of **The New England Journal of Medicine** *. . ."* See Jerome Kassirer and Marcia Angell, "Losing Weight—An Ill-Fated New Year's Resolution," *New Engl J Med* 338, 52–54 (1998).

"Even quite fat people have better health, on average, than fashionably thin women." See the epidemiological studies cited in the notes to Chapter 1. Almost invariably, people with BMI figures below 18.5 have shorter average life expectancies than people with BMI figures in the mid-30s. (An average-height woman with a BMI of 18 weighs 106 pounds; a woman of the same height with a BMI of 35 weighs 202 pounds.) Nearly all fashion models, and most prominent actresses, have BMI figures below 18.5. Obesity researchers try to explain away such awkward facts, when they address them at all, by assuming reverse causation in regard to thinness and ill health, and direct causation in regard to fatness and ill health. In other words, they assume that thin people are thin because they are sick, and that fat people are sick because they are fat. Yet the correlation (unusually thin people not living as long as quite fat people) remains even when researchers go to great lengths to exclude already-sick individuals from their data pools, by, for example, excluding from the study's data everyone who dies within a year or two of entering the study.

"At bottom, journalists tend to believe what they believe about fat because what they believe about fat simply reflects the views about fat held by the people they know best . . ." For liberal and conservative accounts of how the ethnography of journalism affects the framing of public issues, see, respectively, Martin Lee and Norman Solomon, *Unreliable Sources: A Guide to Detecting Bias in News Media* (1990), and Brent Bozell and Brent H. Baker, *And That's the Way It Isn't: A Reference Guide to Media Bias* (1990).

"Recent news reports indicate that fat anxiety is becoming common among six- to eight-year-olds . . ." This anxiety is soon transformed into action. Nearly half of all nine- to eleven-year-old American girls report they are "sometimes or very often" on a diet, and more than half report they feel better about themselves when they are dieting. See "Smaller and Smaller: Eating Disorders Are Now Striking Younger Girls," *Providence Journal-Bulletin* February 16, 2003. In November 2003, the 12-year-old daughter of a colleague performed an experiment at two Boulder supermarkets. Naturally slim, she donned a (very convincing) "fat suit" to solicit donations for the Humane Society while "obese," and then did so again at her natural weight. In each of the four trials, she solicited the donations until exactly 100 people had walked by. She collected a total of $41.05 while thin, and $5.30 while fat.

"In his book The Anatomy of Disgust *. . ."* William Ian Miller, *The Anatomy of Disgust* (1997), p. 36.

"Studies investigating the relationship between weight and health among African American women have found no correlation between increasing weight and mortality among such women . . ." See, for example, Wienpahl et al., "Body Mass Index and 15-year Mortality in a Cohort of Black Men and Women," *J Clin Epidemiol*, 43, 949–60 (1990). See also Fontaine et al., "Years of Life Lost to Obesity," cited in the notes to Chapter 1.

"In his studies of the comparative development of cultures, Jared Diamond . . ." See Jared Diamond, *Guns, Germs and Steel: The Fates of Human Societies* (1999).

Chapter 4

"Indeed, to utter the word 'fat' has become arguably more transgressive . . ." The semantics of the war on fat are significant in themselves. Those who wish to treat fat as a disease assiduously avoid the word, preferring instead to refer to "obesity" or "overweight." In theory, "obesity" could be a neutral descriptive term, defining a particular level of body mass; in practice, it has come to be synonymous with what is defined as a pathological condition. That is why fat activists insist on using the word "fat," which they want to see treated in the same way we treat terms such as "brown-haired" or "freckled." See, for example, Marilyn Wann, *Fat!So?* (1998) at 18: "When you claim the word *fat*, no one can use it against you ever again."

"Between the many varieties of vegetarianism . . ." See Anthony Bourdain, *Kitchen Confidential: Adventures in the Culinary Underbelly* (2001).

"The reason we are getting fatter while eating less fat is that, as Richard Klein points out . . ." See generally, Richard Klein, *Eat Fat* (1996). Relative caloric percentages from fat are taken from the United States Department of Agriculture statistics. See the USDA's website at www.usda.gov.

"Surveys indicate that dieters . . ." For statistics on the number of Americans who are currently trying to lose or not gain weight, see Serdula et al., "Prevalence of Attempting Weight Loss and Strategies for Controlling Weight," *JAMA* 282, 1353–58 (1999).

"We are a nation of dieters, and therefore a nation of snackers . . ." For a discussion of the so-called French paradox (France has one-quarter the obesity rate of the United States, despite a much higher-fat diet) see Rozin et al., "The Ecology of Eating," *Psychol Sci* 14, 450 (2003).

"Laura Fraser describes the phenomenon well . . ." See Fraser, *Losing It*, pp. 118–19.

Chapter 5

"The obituary itself is a fascinating document . . ." See *New York Times*, June 5, 2000, Section A, p. 27.

"Consider the implications of the fact that several studies have found that short men . . ." See Allebeck et al., "Height, Body Mass Index, and Mortality: Do Social Factors Explain the Association?" *Public Health* 106 375–82 (1992); Peck and Vagero, "Adult Body Height, Self-perceived Health and Mortality in the Swedish Population," *J Epidemiol* 43, 380–84 (1984).

"Race and obesity both illustrate how the social effects of an idea can be very real . . ." Perhaps the most interesting parallel to early twenty-first-century obesity studies is provided by mid-nineteenth-century phrenology. Phrenologists operated on the basis of a fundamentally mistaken theory about the meaningfulness of variations in cranial features. Nevertheless, phrenology was for many decades an eminently respectable science, which produced learned journals, scholarly conferences, and endowed professorships. The decline of the field, in the face of ever-growing amounts of empirical disconfirmation, was slowed by the—sometimes explicit but more often implicit—belief that it simply wasn't possible that a well-organized form of scientific knowledge could be based on a fundamental theoretical mistake. See Pierre Schlag, "Law and Phrenology," *Harvard Law Rev*, 110, 887 (1997).

"According to Tony Gardner . . ." See *The New Yorker*, "Thy Neighbor's Fat Suit," July 16, 2001, p. 28.

"Paltrow's own experiences while making the film are revealing." See *The Edmonton Sun*, "Paltrow Puts Hollywood Obsessions to the Test," November 4, 2001, p. SE5.

"A recent essay in the New Yorker . . ." See "Thy Neighbor's Fat Suit," cited above.

"Researchers point out (correctly) that fat people face discrimination . . ." An excellent summary of the available research on discrimination against fat people is Puhl and Brownell, "Bias, Discrimination, and Obesity," *Obesity Res* 9, 788–805. Kelly Brownell's evident empathy for the deep discrimination fat people face has not stopped him from making the quest to turn fat people into thin people the prime focus of his work. See, for example, his book *Food Fight* (2003).

"One University of Arizona study found . . ." Parker et al., "Body Images and Weight Concerns Among African-American and White Adolescent Females," *Human Org* 54, 103–114 (1995).

"Is it a coincidence that black women are both far less obsessed with weight than white women . . ." See, for example, Dacosta and Wilson, "Food Preferences and Eating Attitudes in Three Generations of Black and White Women," *Appetite* (1999), at 183–91; Greenberg and Laporte, "Racial Differences in Body Type Preferences of Men and Women," *J Eating Dis* 19, 275–78 (1996).

"In recent years, companies such as Weight Watchers and Jenny Craig . . ." Fraser, *Losing It*, p. 142–43.

"As for obesity researchers, a recent article noted that black girls have better body images ..." Kemper et al., "Black and White Females' Perceptions of Ideal Body Size and Social Norms," *Obesity Res*, 2, 117–25 (1994).

Chapter 6

"Studies indicate that, when women are asked to estimate the dimensions of their hips and thighs ..." Ben-Touim et al., "Body Size Estimates: Body Image or Body Attitude Measures," *Int J Eating Dis* 9, 57–67 (1990); Galgan and Mable, "Body Satisfaction in College Women: A Survey of Facial and Body Size Components," *Coll Student J* 20, 326–28 (1986).

"Interestingly, some of the studies that indicate women consistently overestimate their actual body size also suggest men prefer women ..." Jacobi and Cash, "In Pursuit of the Perfect Appearance: Discrepancies Among Self-Ideal Precepts of Multiple Physical Attributes," *J Appl Soc Psychol* 24, 379–96 (1994).

"Where, I wonder, are the mainstream feminist organizations ..." See Chapter Seventeen for a discussion of the feminist movement's mixed record movement on issues of body oppression.

"Yet his campaign advisers emphasized to him that he needed to lose 30 pounds ..." A recent *New Yorker* profile of Gore illustrates how we are becoming increasingly sensitive to superficial issues of appearance when evaluating political figures: "[The crowd] took turns speculating about what clues they'd soon be called upon to interpret. Beard or no beard? Earth tones or dark suit? Fat or thin?" "Impressions of Gore," *New Yorker*, August 18, 2003, p. 42.

"All other things being equal, it is probably healthier for an average-height woman to weigh 135 rather than 115 pounds ..." For white women, the low point in the mortality curve tends to be at around a BMI of 24 (140 pounds for an average-height woman). For African American women, the lowest mortality point correlating with weight is about 15 to 20 pounds higher than that. See the studies cited in Chapter 1 for examples.

"There is nothing unusual about these hypothetical examples: as we shall see ..." See Chapter 14 for a discussion of medical studies demonstrating that exactly the same levels of caloric intake and physical activity lead to vast differences in body mass among different individuals.

Chapter 7

For further details regarding Anamarie Regino's family's battle with New Mexico's public health and legal systems, see "Growing Pains," *Denver Post*, August 5, 2001, p. I-01; "Watching Her Weight," *New York Times*, July 8, 2001, at Sec. 6, p. 30; "Feeling Betrayed," *Dallas Morning News*, April 19, 2001, p. 1A; "Parents of Obese Child Say State Abused Its Power by Taking Custody," *St. Louis Post-Dispatch*, February 4, 2001, p. 3A; "Adela Martinez and Margaret Martinez Talk About Anamarie Regino's Obesity," ABC News, *Good Morning America*, June 18, 2001 (transcript).

Chapter 8

"Unfortunately, in modern American journalism, even the best regarded media sources ..." For example, between September of 2001 and September of 2003, the supposed "fact" that fat kills three hundred thousand Americans per year

was cited more than 1,700 times in the major English-language media, in the face of numerous demonstrations that this claim is at best a wild exaggeration, if not a completely spurious piece of junk science.

"Given this, consider the implications of the following piece of reportage . . ." "Study Finds Diet, Exercise and Drug Prevent Diabetes," *Wall Street Journal*, August 8, 2001, p. 1.

"The study followed more than three thousand volunteers for at least three years." Tuomilehto et al., "Prevention of Type 2 Diabetes Mellitus by Changes in Lifestyle Among Subjects with Impaired Glucose Tolerance," *New Engl J Med* 344, 1343–50 (2001). For other studies indicating that lifestyle changes rather than weight loss per se are key to preventing and treating Type 2 diabetes, see Lamarche et al., "Is Body Fat Loss a Determinant Factor in the Improvement of Carbohydrate and Lipid Metabolism Following Aerobic Exercise Training in Obese Women?" *Metabolism* 41, 1249–56 (1992); Barnard et al., "Diet and Exercise in the Treatment of NIDDM," *Diabetes Care* 17, 1469–72 (1994); Diabetes Prevention Program Research Group, "Reduction in the Incidence of Type 2 Diabetes with Lifestyle Intervention or Metformin," *New Engl J Med* 346, 393–403 (2002).

Chapter 9

"In his study of Spanish life in the 1960s . . ." See James Michener, *Iberia* (1968).

"In the film version the character of Bridget Jones is played by a conventionally slim actress . . ." Zellweger has since agreed to gain back the same 20 pounds for a sequel to the film. It was widely noted that she will be paid $100,000 per extra pound to play the role of a "fat" 129-pound woman.

"For obvious reasons advertisers and their clients would like to condition men to become as neurotic about their appearance . . ." See "Holding Back the Years," *Financial Times*, August 16, 2003, p. 6.

"Recognizing the fundamental fraudulence of the war on fat . . ." Brad Pitt has a reported BMI of 27.5, which puts him squarely in the middle of the "overweight" range, according to our public health authorities. Paltrow, on the other hand, has a BMI of 16, which correlates with a far higher degree of epidemiological risk than all but the most extreme levels of obesity.

Chapter 10

"Consider this passage from Roberta Seid's invaluable history . . ." Roberta Seid, *Never Too Thin: Why Women Are at War with Their Bodies* (1989), pp. 120–21.

"This is the theoretical mechanism behind the empirical fact that dieters often end up weighing more . . ." An article in the October 2003 issue of the medical journal *Pediatrics* reports that at any one time around a quarter of all American children between the ages of nine and fourteen report they are dieting, and that the dieting children gain more weight than children who report they do not diet. The authors speculate that this may be a product of either the slowing of the metabolism produced by chronic dieting, or binge behavior when the children find themselves unable to diet perpetually, or a combination of these factors.

" 'Someone needs to say that the emperor has no clothes,' says Wayne Callaway . . ." See Fraser, *Losing It*, p. 229.

"Do these researchers actually believe American culture is too tolerant toward fat?" As counterintuitive as this thesis might seem, it is put forth with increasing

frequency in both the medical and popular literature. For a striking example, see Greg Critser's book *Fat Land* (2002), which argues that Americans are fat because, among other reasons, the media elites fail to convey to the masses that slimness is socially desirable. Or consider this quote from a prominent obesity researcher: "People don't realize that they're fat . . . There are so many fat Americans now that it's sometimes the thin ones that are in the minority." Quoted in Saguy and Riley, "Fat Attack: Scientific and Political Debates over Obesity" (forthcoming).

"But let us take those crude statistics on their face." See the numerous epidemiological studies discussed in Chapter 1 for statistical breakdowns of the effects of "overweight" and "underweight" on life expectancy.

" 'Like cinema starlets who have only recently been manufactured . . .' " Frederick Exley, *A Fan's Notes* (1968), pp. 384–85.

Chapter 11

"According to the U.S. federal government, Marshall Faulk is obese." I calculated BMI figures for all of the league's more than 1,500 players by employing the statistics provided by the rosters of NFL teams, as listed on their official websites, in the summer of 2001.

"Indeed, some proponents of the BMI tables have begun to admit this indirectly . . ." See, for example, the National Institutes of Health website (www. nih.gov), which acknowledges that "some very muscular people may fall into the overweight category when they are actually healthy and fit." The public health establishment's manipulation of the BMI tables in this regard is essentially a verbal shell game. When confronted with the fact that many people who by every objective measure are in superb physical condition are also "overweight" and "obese" according to the BMI charts, public health officials admit that the charts are meaningless in such situations. Yet this admission is instantly forgotten when these same officials declare that, according to these same charts, nearly two-thirds of adult Americans are "overweight" and "obese."

"In their comprehensive review of the literature, Paul Ernsberger and Paul Haskew . . ." Ernsberger and Haskew, "Health Implications of Obesity: An Alternative View," *J Obesity W Reg* 6, 67 (1987).

"Yet only around 30 percent of the population qualifies for even this modest standard." This figure is a rough estimate, based on data from public health surveys, and studies such as those conducted by the Cooper Institute (cited in Chapter 1). One consequence of the fact that until recently the medical establishment took little notice of the importance of activity to health is that relatively little solid data exists regarding the activity levels of Americans, and how those levels relate to body mass.

"Wann sums up the principles of the nascent fat fitness movement . . ." Marilyn Wann, *Fat!So?* (1998), p. 61.

Chapter 12

"As Glenn Gaesser has put it, 'Of all our convictions about health . . .' " Gaesser, *Big Fat Lies* (2002), p. 83.

"Perhaps the best evidence that people trying to lose weight are not motivated primarily by health concerns . . ." According to the Centers for Disease Control and Prevention, 70 percent of all "overweight" American women are attempting to

lose weight at any particular time, as opposed to around 50 percent of "ideal weight" women. Significantly more women than men are dieting; the average American woman has a BMI of about 25; and rates of dieting peak around the age of forty. Thus the average American dieter is a middle-aged woman with a BMI in the mid-to-high 20s.

"A typical set of statistics from a large-scale epidemiological study . . ." Waaler et al., "Height, Weight and Mortality: The Norwegian Experience," *Acta Med Scanda Suppl* 679, 1–56 (1984).

"A few years ago, **Esquire** *magazine conducted a survey . . ."* *Esquire,* February 1994, p. 73.

"It becomes easier to understand that preference when considering such data as that provided by a recent university study . . ." See *Texas Monthly,* January 1997, p. 106.

Chapter 13

"Austin's web page makes it even clearer . . ." See www.secure.deniseaustin.com.

"Consider the classic symptoms of anorexia . . ." These descriptions are taken from the *Diagnostic and Statistical Manual of Mental Disorders,* Fourth Edition, (DSM-IV).

"Despite a mass of epidemiological evidence that, in the words of one of the world's most eminent obesity experts . . ." Ancel Keys, *Seven Countries: A Multivariate Analysis of Death and Coronary Heart Disease* (1980).

"When someone such as Britney Spears . . ." Quoted in *The Observer,* September 16, 2001, p. 10.

"Over the course of the last century, what has been considered the ideal body weight for American women . . ." See, generally, Seid, *Never Too Thin;* Schwartz, *Never Satisfied;* Fraser, *Losing It;* Klein, *Eat Fat;* Chernin, *The Obsession.*

"By way of comparison, although today we remember flapper fashion as being focused on boyish thinness . . ." Seid, *Never Too Thin,* p. 97.

"Anyone familiar with what Naomi Wolf has characterized as 'the cult of dieting' . . ." Naomi Wolf's *The Beauty Myth* is an essential text for anyone who wishes to understand the ideological underpinnings and political consequences of America's weight obsession. Consider the following: "Dieting is the most potent political sedative in women's history; a quietly mad population is a tractable one."

"America's dieters, like Kafka's hunger artist . . ." See Kafka, *Collected Stories* (1993), p. 209.

Chapter 14

"For most people, the standard prescriptions for losing weight do not work . . ." Some statistics on dieting patterns among contemporary Americans, from Serdula et al., "Prevalence of Attempting Weight Loss and Strategies for Controlling Weight," *JAMA* 282, 1353–58 (1999). Among people with BMIs under 25, 8.6 percent of men and 28.7 percent of women are dieting. Among those with BMIs between 25 and 30, 35.7 percent of men and 59.6 percent of women are dieting. Among those with BMIs of 30 and higher, 60.4 percent of men and 70.1 percent of women are dieting. This is a snapshot of the percentages at a particular moment: The percentages of people who spend significant amounts of time dieting in each of these weight cohorts is undoubtedly much higher. Note that the percentage of dieters correlates very

strongly with increasing weight, and that at any one time the vast majority of obese persons are dieting. It is clear that fatness causes dieting. It is also clear that dieting causes fatness. The denial of the second point may be the single most crucial feature of the obesity myth.

"Specifically, a growing number of obesity researchers, eating disorder specialists . . ." The Health at Every Size movement features a diverse group of proponents. Many of the leading figures have some association with the *Healthy Weight Journal*, a peer-reviewed medical journal, published by BL Decker, which in January 2004 was renamed *Health at Every Size*. The journal is edited by Jonathan Robison and Wayne Miller. Its editorial board includes Joanne Ikeda, Debby Burgard, Glenn Gaesser, Paul Ernsberger, Marilyn Wann, Karin Kratina, Patricia Lyons, Frances Berg, Lynn MacAfee, Lisa Tealer, and Karen Petersmarck. All these people have published extensively on the subject of weight and health, from a HAES point of view. The most comprehensive explanation and defense of the HAES approach is found in Gaesser's invaluable book *Big Fat Lies* (2002). Jon Robison maintains a website dedicated to HAES, which offers an excellent introduction to the subject, along with much bibliographical information. See www.jonrobison.net/size.html.

"The HAES movement itself is based on three core principles . . ." Robison, "Health at Every Size: Antidote for the Obesity Epidemic," *Healthy Weight J* 17(2) (2003).

"For instance, HAES proponents aim to publicize medical studies demonstrating that people who ingest exactly the same number of calories . . ." See Bouchard et al., "The Response to Long-Term Overfeeding in Identical Twins" *New Engl J Med* 322, 1477–82 (1990).

"Similarly, a 1999 study published in Science . . ." Levine et al., "Role of Non-Exercise Activity Thermogenesis (NEAT) in Resistance to Fat Gain in Humans," *Science* 283, 212–14 (1999).

"The movement's seven 'principles for medical practice' are . . ." See Robison, cited above.

"As Glenn Gaesser points out . . ." Gaesser, *Big Fat Lies*, p. 83.

"For example, Linda Bacon, a nutrition researcher at the University of California-Davis . . ." Bacon et al., "Effects of Supporting 'Health at Every Size' and Intuitive Eating for Obese Female Chronic Dieters: A Randomized Clinical Trial," (forthcoming).

Chapter 15

"Three years later Chambrin revealed that he believed the first lady got rid of him because he was too fat . . ." Washington Times, September 9, 1997, p. A1.

"According to Clinton's people, Chambrin was fired not because he was fat . . ." Memphis Commercial Appeal, September 14, 1997, p. A7.

"Indeed, a woman of considerably greater importance in Bill Clinton's life . . ." Joyce Milton, *The First Partner: Hillary Rodham Clinton* (1999), p. 70.

"In a touch straight out of Faulkner, the only person in Bill's immediate family . . ." The First Partner, p. 71.

" 'Look, I want you to know that I've had it up to here with beauty queens . . .' " The First Partner, p. 72.

" 'This is fun. Women are throwing themselves at me.' " James B. Stewart, *Blood Sport: The President and His Adversaries* (1996), p. 70.

" '*It was such a sweet moment. It was the first time I had seen him without a shirt . . .*' " Andrew Morton, *Monica's Story* (1999), p. 66.

" '*I saw you in the hall today—you looked really skinny.*' " *Monica's Story*, p. 72.

"*Monica's teenage years were dominated by the devastation being a 'fat' girl at Beverly Hills High wrought . . .*" *Monica's Story*, pp. 30–42.

" '*Her relationship with Andy [Blieler] was damaging to her . . .*" *Monica's Story*, p. 49.

" '*She always saw herself as second best in her relationships with men . . .*' " *Monica's Story*, p. 64.

"*Twenty years older than Monica, Tripp had been teased mercilessly . . .*" *Monica's Story*, pp. 92–93.

"*Something else that has become clear with hindsight is that Tripp was obsessed with Bill Clinton . . .*" *Monica's Story*, p. 95.

"*It was at this juncture, in the fall of 1997, that the weight obsessions of two of the principal actors in the scandal . . .*" *Monica's Story*, pp. 143–44.

"*A 'fat cheesy slut' was one particularly vicious description . . .*" *The Star*, October 10, 1998.

"*Monica Lewinsky embodied, at a deep level of social anxiety, a sort of reincarnation of the rapacious, sexually insatiable Jewess . . .*" For an interesting discussion of parallels between weight prejudice and anti-Semitism, see W. Charisse Goodman, *The Invisible Woman: Confronting Weight Prejudice in America* (1995).

Chapter 16

"*The Lewinsky affair soon propelled her to the position of alpha female among a bevy of telegenic right-wing commentators . . .*" For an amusing discussion of pundettes, see Michelle Cottle, "Washington Diarist," *The New Republic*, July 10, 2000, p. 48: "Most producers deny that appearance plays a big part in whom they book. This is a fib on the magnitude of 'I did not have sexual relations with that woman.' "

"*In the words of another pundette, Heather Nauert . . .*" *Washington Post*, May 25, 2000, p. C01.

All quotes attributed to Estrich are from Susan Estrich, *Making the Case for Yourself: A Diet Book for Smart Women* (1998).

"*Third, remarkably for a self-identified feminist, Estrich never notes the obvious political implications of the common theme that links the times in her life when she was least able to diet . . .*" In regard to the feminist literature which links dieting with gender oppression, Estrich comments: "I read all the popular books by beautiful feminists that were supposed to convince you that being slim and beautiful is just some sexist man's fantasy, but frankly, on me the books failed. They don't liberate me. I don't look in the mirror and smile at my stomach. I don't feel better about my body. I just feel vain, foolish, and stupid in addition to fat."

"*At least Estrich admits that, in the context of what Naomi Wolf has termed the cult of dieting . . .*" See, generally, Naomi Wolf, *The Beauty Myth* (1991).

"*Coulter has even complained recently that she can't get a date . . .*" *The Guardian*, May 17, 2003, p. 14.

Chapter 17

"Perhaps my favorite single example of how much of the work in this field is an embarrassment to the word 'science'..." Drenick et al., "Prolonged Starvation as Treatment for Severe Obesity," *JAMA* 187, 100–5 (1964).

"As two leading dissenters in the obesity research community have put it..." Ernsberger and Haskew, "Health Implications of Obesity: An Alternative View," *J Obesity W Reg* 6, 67 (1987).

"As Karl Popper first pointed out more than seventy years ago..." Karl Popper, *The Logic of Scientific Discovery* (1959). Other classic discussions of this point include Thomas Kuhn, *The Structure of Scientific Revolutions* (1970), and Paul Feyerabend, *Against Method* (1993).

"I have yet to find a dress larger than size 12..." I've been told that many fashionable boutiques in New York City do not carry any merchandise above size 8.

"Here again we have a social and economic puzzle: a group of retailers whose products fail completely to intersect with the needs of half the potential market..." See "Sizing Up the Marketplace," *Chicago Sun Times,* July 8, 2003, p. 40.

"Individual feminists, such as Naomi Wolf and Susan Bordo, have written devastating critiques..." See Naomi Wolf, *The Beauty Myth* (1991); Susan Bordo, *Unbearable Weight: Feminism, Western Culture, and the Body* (1995).

"Such groups have been almost completely silent about the far greater levels of discrimination so-called obese women in particular face..." I am grateful to Abigail Saguy for pointing this out to me, and for helping me clarify my thinking on the complex issue of feminist organizations and fat discrimination.

"That is why much of the most powerful criticism of those ideals has not come from feminists in size 6 dresses..." See Marilyn Wann, *Fat!So?* (1998); Sondra Solovay, *Tipping the Scales of Justice: Fighting Weight-Based Discrimination* (2000); Carol Wiley (ed.), *Journeys to Self-Acceptance: Fat Women Speak* (1994). Jennifer Portnick is the San Francisco area aerobics instructor who brought a successful complaint under the city's nondiscrimination ordinance, against a Jazzercise health club franchise, for discriminating against her because of her weight. See *San Francisco Chronicle,* May 7, 2002, p. A1.

"The emotions fat elicits are fraught with the classic features produced by that which disgusts us..." See, generally, William Ian Miller, *The Anatomy of Disgust* (1997).

"In his famous essay 'Protestant Asceticism and the Spirit of Capitalism'..." See Runciman, ed., *Weber: Selections in Translation* (1978), pp. 138–73.

"As Greg Critser notes, 'in upscale corporate America, being fat is a sure-fire career-killer.'" Greg Critser, "Let Them Eat Fat," *Harper's,* March 2000, p. 42.

" 'I hate to say it, but if you have this gene you can smoke and you can be fat...' " *The New York Times,* October 15, 2003, p. A16.

"Americans worry, with good reason, that we have become too big for our own good..." Cf. Tony Judt, "Anti-Americans Abroad," *New York Review of Books,* May 1, 2003: "If you want to understand how America appears to the world today, consider the sport-utility vehicle. Oversized and overweight, the SUV disdains negotiated agreements to restrict atmospheric pollution. It consumes inordinate quantities of scarce resources to furnish its privileged inhabitants with supererogatory services. It exposes outsiders to deadly risk in order to provide for the illusory security of its occupants. In a crowded world, the SUV appears as a dangerous anachro-

nism. Like U.S. foreign policy, the sport-utility vehicle comes packaged in sonorous mission statements; but underneath it is just an oversized pickup truck with too much power."

"As long ago as the 1950s, marketing analyst Victor Lebow pointed out . . ." Quoted in Michael F. Jacobson and Laurie Ann Mazur, *Marketing Madness: A Survival Guide for a Consumer Society* (1995), p. 191.

"Indeed, as UCLA sociologist Abigail Saguy suggested to me . . ." Saguy has undertaken a long-term research project to study the social construction of "obesity" as a health and/or political issue in contemporary America. See, for example, Saguy and Riley, "Fat Attack: Scientific and Political Debates over Obesity" (forthcoming).

" 'Moral panic' is a term coined by Stanley Cohen in the 1960s . . ." See Stanley Cohen, *Folk Devils and Moral Panics* (2002).

"American history is rich with examples of moral panics." On the drug war, see Michael Massing, *The Fix* (2000). On sexual abuse in schools and day care centers, see Dorothy Rabinowitz, *No Crueler Tyrannies: Accusation, False Witness, and Other Terrors of Our Times* (2003). On McCarthyism, see Albert Fried, ed., *The Great American Red Scare* (1996). For a superb sociological analysis of various exaggerated and irrational fears in contemporary America, see Barry Glassner, *The Culture of Fear: Why Americans Are Afraid of the Wrong Things* (1999). Absurdly, apologists for the drug war, McCarthyism, etc., often insist their opponents are claiming that drugs are harmless, that there were no communist agents in the American government in the 1950s, and that there is no such thing as sexual abuse of preschool children. The parallel argument in the war on fat is the absurd assertion that those who question any aspect of that war are claiming that "obesity" is completely benign.

"Anorexia has a higher fatality rate than any other mental illness." The National Association of Anorexia and Associated Disorders estimates that the fatality rate from the syndrome may be as high as 15 percent—several times higher than that associated with major depression.

"In her pursuit of virtue, she becomes a secularized shadow of the so-called holy anorexics of premodern Europe . . ." See Rudolph M. Bell, *Holy Anorexia* (1987).

Chapter 18

"Near the end of his essay 'Why I Write' George Orwell . . ." Ian Angus and Sonia Orwell, eds., *George Orwell: An Age Like This 1920–1940: The Collected Essays, Journalism & Letters* (1968), p. 3.

"When I began to write this book I was fat." As Abigail Saguy and Kevin Riley point out, a routine tactic of the war on fat involves referring to the bodies of the opponents of that war in order to discredit those opponents: "Obesity researchers [are] more likely to evoke the bodies of fat acceptance activists to discredit them than to do this for Health At Every Size scholars, partly because many leading HAES scholars . . . are thin men. In fact, Glenn Gaesser said in an interview that his book editor only agreed to publish *Big Fat Lies* when she saw that he was tall and thin because she reasoned that, if he had been fat, the book 'would have been viewed as almost a rationalization for being fat, [as if he had] a personal axe to grind.' [By contrast] most fat activists are women who would be categorized as morbidly obese. In interviews, obesity researchers suggested that this fact . . . discredited them as simply making excuses for their weight. That a fat person is incapable of speaking *objectively* about weight seems to be readily accepted, while the idea that a thin

person would be biased in a different but equally strong direction seems to be less intuitive. In this case, thinness functions as an 'unmarked category,' much as whiteness or maleness are considered unmarked categories for race and gender, respectively. In all of these cases, the biases of the dominant group are ignored." Saguy and Riley, "Fat Attack: Scientific and Political Debates over Obesity" (forthcoming).

This perceptive analysis implies that the ideal of interpretive objectivity may be even less attainable in the context of a psychologically and politically fraught issue such as weight than it is in regard to most other medical and public health controversies. It follows that, while there is nothing necessarily illegitimate about suggesting that many fat activists hold the views they do, in part, because they are fat, it is also legitimate to suggest that many people who are actively involved in prosecuting the war on fat do so, in part, because of psychological investments they have made in what they see as the medical and/or moral significance of their own thinness. This is no doubt especially the case among people who have lost weight, and wish to ascribe moral value to that fact.

Body Mass Index Table

Height (inches)	BMI 19	20	21	22	23	24	25	26	27	28	29	30	31	32	33	34	35	36	37	38	39	40	41	42	43	44	45	46	47	48	49	50	51	52	53	54
																	Body Weight (pounds)																			
58	91	96	100	105	110	115	119	124	129	134	138	143	148	153	158	162	167	172	177	181	186	191	196	201	205	210	215	220	224	229	234	239	244	248	253	258
59	94	99	104	109	114	119	124	128	133	138	143	148	153	158	163	168	173	178	183	188	193	198	203	208	212	217	222	227	232	237	242	247	252	257	262	267
60	97	102	107	112	118	123	128	133	138	143	148	153	158	163	168	174	179	184	189	194	199	204	209	215	220	225	230	235	240	245	250	255	261	266	271	276
61	100	106	111	116	122	127	132	137	143	148	153	158	164	169	174	180	185	190	195	201	206	211	217	222	227	232	238	243	248	254	259	264	269	275	280	285
62	104	109	115	120	126	131	136	142	147	153	158	164	169	175	180	186	191	196	202	207	213	218	224	229	235	240	246	251	256	262	267	273	278	284	289	295
63	107	113	118	124	130	135	141	146	152	158	163	169	174	180	186	191	197	203	208	214	220	225	231	237	242	248	254	259	265	270	278	282	287	293	299	304
64	110	116	122	128	134	140	145	151	157	163	169	174	180	186	192	197	204	209	215	221	227	232	238	244	250	256	262	267	273	279	285	291	296	302	308	314
65	114	120	126	132	138	144	150	156	162	168	174	180	186	192	198	204	210	216	222	228	234	240	246	252	258	264	270	276	282	288	294	300	306	312	318	324
66	118	124	130	136	142	148	155	161	167	173	179	186	192	198	204	210	216	223	229	235	241	247	253	260	266	272	278	284	291	297	303	309	315	322	328	334
67	121	127	134	140	146	153	159	166	172	178	185	191	198	204	211	217	223	230	236	242	249	255	261	268	274	280	287	293	299	306	312	319	325	331	338	344
68	125	131	138	144	151	158	164	171	177	184	190	197	203	210	216	223	230	236	243	249	256	262	269	276	282	289	295	302	308	315	322	328	335	341	348	354
69	128	135	142	149	155	162	169	176	182	189	196	203	209	216	223	230	236	243	250	257	263	270	277	284	291	297	304	311	318	324	331	338	345	351	358	365
70	132	139	146	153	160	167	174	181	188	195	202	209	216	222	229	236	243	250	257	264	271	278	285	292	299	306	313	320	327	334	341	348	355	362	369	376
71	136	143	150	157	165	172	179	186	193	200	208	215	222	229	236	243	250	257	265	272	279	286	293	301	308	315	322	329	338	343	351	358	365	372	379	386
72	140	147	154	162	169	177	184	191	199	206	213	221	228	235	242	250	258	265	272	279	287	294	302	309	316	324	331	338	346	353	361	368	375	383	390	397
73	144	151	159	166	174	182	189	197	204	212	219	227	235	242	250	257	265	272	280	288	295	302	310	318	325	333	340	348	355	363	371	378	386	393	401	408
74	148	155	163	171	179	186	194	202	210	218	225	233	241	249	256	264	272	280	287	295	303	311	319	326	334	342	350	358	365	373	381	389	396	404	412	420
75	152	160	168	176	184	192	200	208	216	224	232	240	248	256	264	272	279	287	295	303	311	319	327	335	343	351	359	367	375	383	391	399	407	415	423	431
76	156	164	172	180	189	197	205	213	221	230	238	246	254	263	271	279	287	295	304	312	320	328	336	344	353	361	369	377	385	394	402	410	418	426	435	443

Source: Adapted from *Clinical Guidelines on the Identification, Evaluation, and Treatment of Overweight and Obesity in Adults: The Evidence Report.*

Suggestions for Further Reading

This book's endnotes reference only a small part of the extensive literature criticizing the science, culture, and politics of America's obsession with weight. The following books are essential reading for anyone who wishes to understand the full extent of that obsession.

Susan Bordo, *Unbearable Weight: Feminism, Western Culture, and the Body* (1995).

Kim Chernin, *The Obsession: Reflections on the Tyranny of Slenderness* (1981).

Laura Fraser, *Losing It: False Hopes and Fat Profits in the Diet Industry* (1998).

Glenn Gaesser, *Big Fat Lies: The Truth About Your Weight and Your Health* (2002).

Richard Klein, *Eat Fat* (1996).

Susie Orbach, *Fat Is a Feminist Issue* (1978).

Hillel Schwartz, *Never Satisfied: A Cultural History of Diets, Fantasies and Fat* (1986).

Roberta Seid, *Never Too Thin: Why Women Are at War with Their Bodies* (1989).

Marilyn Wann, *Fat!So?* (1999).

Naomi Wolf, *The Beauty Myth: How Images of Beauty Are Used Against Women* (1991).

Acknowledgments

This book would not have been possible without the cooperation of hundreds of people who agreed to be interviewed about their experiences with food, dieting, body image, and related topics. Parts or all of some of these interviews appear in the book (I have changed names, and, in a few cases, unessential biographical details).

Paul Ernsberger and Glenn Gaesser were extraordinarily generous in sharing their medical expertise with me. Each answered dozens of questions over the course of many months, and helped clarify a great number of issues posed by a voluminous and complex scientific literature.

Jean Braithwaite, Melissa Hart, Mimi Wesson, and Steve Williams read and critiqued an early version of the manuscript. Their suggestions were very useful to the process of revising it. So were those made by the late Jed Mattes, who contributed much to this project in various ways. I wish he could have seen this book.

My friend and colleague Sarah Krakoff believed in this project from the beginning, and gave its author a great deal of intellectual, editorial, and emotional support. This book could not have been written without her help.

Abigail Saguy provided a detailed and immensely useful critique of the manuscript, and shared various insights regarding the framing of obesity as a social concept that had a crucial impact on the book's final form. She has contributed greatly to my understanding of the sociological aspects of this subject—which is to say to all aspects of it.

My agent Jim Levine has been indispensable to every step of the book's publication. He performs a job that has more facets than I could have imagined before he undertook the task of selling and helping to publish this book, with an energy and skill he brings to all his projects.

Erin Moore has been the sort of editor every writer hopes to work with. Her passion for this project has been inspirational, and her remarkably deft editing has made this a far better book. My debt to her is profound.

I wish to thank Bill Shinker of Gotham Books for having such excellent taste in editors, manuscripts, and Italian restaurants.

I also want to thank Jon Chait and Chris Orr at *The New Republic*, Marc Miller, Marilyn Wann, Jon Robison, Deb Burgard, Miriam Berg, Francie Berg, Karin Kratina, Jennifer Portnick, Joanne Ikeda, Cindy Dallow, Ellen Shuman, Barbara Bruno, Pat Lyons, Linda Bacon, Sandy Szwarc, and everyone else at Show Me the Data.

Finally, I wish to thank my family for tolerating the birth of another book.

Index